About Face

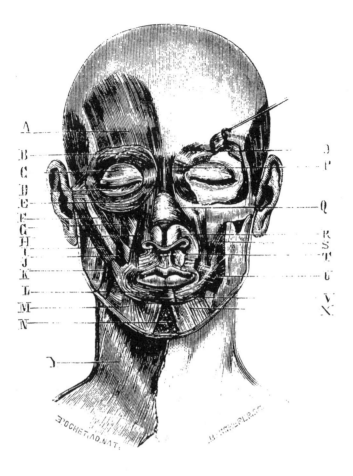

An anatomical preparation of the muscles of the face. Note the way in which certain muscles are ascribed expressive functions. (From G.–B Duchenne de Boulogne, *Mechanisme de la Physiolonomie Humaine ou Analyse Electro-physiologique de l'Expression des Passions*, 1862, republished as *The Mechanism of Human Facial Expression*," Cambridge: Cambridge University Press, 1990. Reprinted with permission.)

About Face

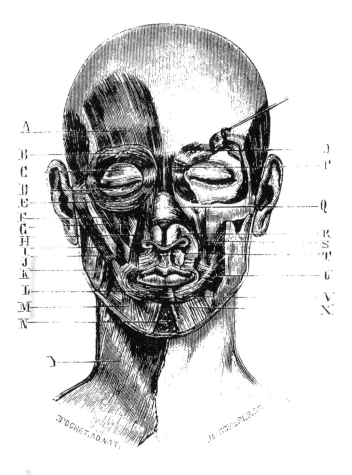

An anatomical preparation of the muscles of the face. Note the way in which certain muscles are ascribed expressive functions. (From G.–B Duchenne de Boulogne, *Mechanisme de la Physiolonomie Humaine ou Analyse Electro-physiologique de l'Expression des Passions*, 1862, republished as *The Mechanism of Human Facial Expression*," Cambridge: Cambridge University Press, 1990. Reprinted with permission.)

About Face

Jonathan Cole

A Bradford Book
The MIT Press
Cambridge, Massachusetts
London, England

This book was set in Bembo on the Miles 33 Typesetting System by Graphic
Composition, Inc. and was printed and bound in the United States of America.

Library of Congress Cataloging-in-Publication Data

Cole, Jonathan David.
  About face/Jonathan Cole
  p. cm.
  "A Bradford book."
  Includes index.
  ISBN O-262–03246-5 (alk. paper)
  1. Facial expression. 2. Face—Movement disorders. I. Title
QP327.C65 1997
612'.92—dc21   97–2099
                                                        CIP

Excerpts from *Nobody Nowhere* by Donna Williams. Copyright © 1992 by Donna
Williams. Reprinted by permission of A.P. Watt Limited on behalf of Donna
Williams; Corgi Books, an imprint of Transworld Publishers Ltd. (UK); Times
Books, a Division of Random House, Inc. (USA); Bantam Doubleday Dell
Transworld Publishers (Australia) Pty Ltd.; and Doubleday Canada Ltd.

Excerpts from *Somebody Somewhere* by Donna Williams. Copyright © 1994 by
Donna Williams. Reprinted by permission of A.P. Watt Limited on behalf of Donna
Williams; Corgi Books, an imprint of Transworld Publishers Ltd. (UK); Times
Books, a Division of Random House, Inc. (USA); Bantam Doubleday Dell
Transworld Publishers (Australia) Pty Ltd.; and Doubleday Canada Ltd.

To those who allowed me to listen, to Oliver who taught me how, and to Sue, of course.

"The human body is the best picture of the human soul."
—Ludwig Wittgenstein, *Philosophical Investigations*, 1953

"I live in the facial expression of the other, as I feel him living in mine . . . "
—Maurice Merleau-Ponty, *The Primacy of Perception*, 1964

Contents

Acknowledgments

Without the subjects whose narratives are contained within this book, the book and its thesis would not have been worthwhile. I was welcomed, often into their homes, and allowed to listen to aspects of their lives and feelings they had previously not disclosed; listening, I felt a sense of responsibility and of privilege. My hope is that I have written as well as the stories deserve. It is to these subjects that I dedicate this book in part.

I am enormously grateful to those professional workers who answered my questions and gave of their time to talk and whose names are within the book. In particular, thanks to Colin Brennan, Linda Anderson, Carmel Briggs, Anthony Collins, Bill Lang, Bencie Woll, James Partridge, John Aspinall, Jim Cronin, Caroline Garland, Peter Hobson, Jane Walker, and Gus McGrowther. Many people have read the book in manuscript and made constructive criticisms. Early on Don Wark, Sue Balfour, Kim McCulloch, George Lloyd-Roberts, Bidi Evans, Marsha Ivins and Emma Crichton-Miller were very helpful in moving the book from ideas and stories to a whole, while being aware of the fragile nature of an author's ego. My secretary, Sue Macey, helped enormously with typing early drafts.

Later, more detailed criticism came from Shaun Gallagher, John Campbell, and Tony Marcel. I thank them for extending my thoughts on the subject and for helping me improve the book. I have been very fortunate in being able to use such penetrating minds. I met all three at a Kings College seminar to which I was invited by Tony Marcel. For this, and for countless acts of kindness, special thanks is due. Most detailed and useful criticism also came from The MIT Press's anonymous reviewers, and my gratitude extends to them too.

At MIT Teri Mendelsohn and Harry Stanton first approached me about writing the book. Fiona Stevens initiated and then Amy Pierce and Katherine Arnoldi brought to completion the editorial aspects. I am enormously grateful to them all.

This study was supported in part by Poole Hospital NHS Trust and I am grateful to Chief Executive Jan Filochowski for his acquiescence to my academic and research interests.

My wife, Sue, and children, Eleanor, Lydia, Celia, and Georgia, suffered my fascination and indeed obsession with matters facial for several years uncomplainingly. Sue acted as sounding board and censor for many embryonic ideas; I have that and much, much more to thank her for.

Lastly, when I first became interested in the face some years ago I wrote to a friend about the subject. As ever, he was sympathetic and intellectually generous and encouraging. Then, a little while later, there arrived a copy of Charles Bell's book on the face in its 1824 edition which he had sent as a gift. Knowing of my love for Bell, for books, and for writing, it was his way of encouraging me to go further in the subject. So it is with Oliver Sacks that I end these acknowledgments and to him that I, in part, dedicate this book.

About Face

The Pre-face: "Tell, Please"

1

Mary

The second case of the neurological demonstration was wheeled into the lecture theatre. She sat on the chair impassively. She looked at our group of neurologists, students, and nurses, some interested, some bored. Before us was an elderly lady; we looked but could not work out how she felt. She seemed anxious and frightened; that much we knew, though it was not clear *how* we knew, for she had lost all facial expression. Her tongue movements and swallowing were also poor; she held a small handkerchief in her hand to wipe her mouth. But what was immediately apparent was the lack of movement in her face. This disturbed us, for we could not gauge if our questions were being received with the sympathy with which they were asked, nor if she was cooperating in answering or even comprehending them.

Mary offered to write her answers down, but time was short. We went onto an examination of her problem in neurological jargon—bilateral seventh nerve paresis, bulbar muscles gone, swallowing reflexes lost, minor weakness in limbs—before thanking her for coming and settling down to discuss her case. It was difficult to localize the lesion, but there appeared to have been ischemic brain damage, widespread and probably bilateral given the rare nature of her condition. Some wondered if she was also slightly demented, given her problem with comprehending and answering us. The frustration shown in her arm gestures gave the lie to that as far as I was concerned, though the group agreed it was a possibility. There was little to offer in the way of treatment; some recovery might occur. Next case.

Opening the Seam

I went away from the meeting and carried on with my work, but continued thinking about Mary. As I wandered around the wards I slowly realized why. I had spent much of my life making judgments about people, creating character from appearance, words, and actions. I thought I had become expert in these constructions, just like everyone else. But Mary's appearance was so impenetrable that I could tell little about her. To be in the presence of someone without facial animation, and so almost without "face," had deprived me of a main discloser of others. Her facial paralysis had left her with no fixed or recognizable expression—that was disquieting enough—but neither could she react visibly to those around her. She brought into question for me the relation between a person's face and his or her personality and self, a relationship so fundamental and "given" that I had never previously doubted or even thought about it.

The doctors had thought her demented not because she could not respond—she had used body language and offered to write her answers down—but because a large part of the response we looked for depended on her face. Without it we had looked straight through her face, interpreting it as the nothingness of dementia. Without a face she as a person was all but invalidated. Her disease had opened a seam between the face and self I had not realized was there.

Of course, like most people, I always looked around on the train, or in public places, not just to track pretty girls, but to study faces. I tried to match faces to character and life history, to mood and type. Whether I succeeded I had little way of knowing, for most of these people I saw but never met. It was a game, but it was also an imperative—it is my nature, it is our nature.

Never having seen a subject without facial expression, and never having considered its medical problems, I asked medical friends and colleagues: they had the same experience—as medical students and doctors we were taught little. I looked at textbooks of medicine and then neurology and ear, nose and throat diseases. Their long indexes contained no mention of facial expression.

All right, I thought, so medicine is about the big things, about fixing cleft palates, about setting broken bones; maybe movement of the face is too intricate to be the concern of mainstream doctors. Maybe disorders of the face are dealt with by specialists in plastic surgery. That seemed plausible and desirable. Yet alterations in facial expression were all about, if only I had focused on them, for instance in neurology, the impassive facies of a man with Parkinson's disease, or in psychiatry, in almost any condition.[1] How was it that it was not looked at more? Maybe the answer was as it had been for Mary, in front of the doctors, that it was disguised by being so obvious.

I began to read psychological accounts of the face, theses on sociology and the work of primate ethologists. Slowly as I read and thought, ideas about facial action formed in my mind. Yet as I explored these ideas I was drawn toward people whose faces had altered their lives. For I felt that their experience was an important way to approach the face, and what it represented, and a way of exploring the relations between the face and personality. Bernstein after all had written that, "it was in disease that an individual reveals his true nature."[2] Not just his nature, I thought, all our natures seemed bound up with our faces in such a way that these individuals might tell us much about ourselves.

This book represents my journey to try to understand the consequences of various losses of face. Like many journeys the way became clear only when I looked back. Wittgenstein said, "Don't think, look." I certainly set out to look and to feel and so to understand what it was like to be "without face." As I did, however, I began to think, and so with this I explore the face by advancing a natural history and theory of the face from scientific work and from the narratives of a series of individuals with unusual faces. In so doing is revealed, I hope, something of our nature and how it is defined, in part, by the face.

In chapter 4, Bone to Brain, I discuss the evolution of the face, from its beginnings as the carrier of the senses (vision and taste) and the opening of gut and lung, seen in amphibians, to the exquisitely mobile and subtle faces of primates and of ourselves. I give a brief account of the mechanics of the face and its perception. Our faces display our individuality, age, sex, mood, and much more than is seen from the head and snouts of lower animals. The development of the face may parallel the evolution of primates and humans, and reveal something about the evolutionary pressures which led to our emergence. I explore this facial evolution in chapter 5, beginning with the work of ethologists. From these studies of behavior in animals emerge ideas about the face as a displayer of behavior.

Such a role for the face, however, leaves little room on our faces for inner feelings. By observation of primates I argue that facial movements in fact are more than predictors of behavior. I talked with someone who left a career as a primate ethologist to become a psychoanalyst. Frustrated by the limitations of studying the behavior of chimpanzees, and by her inability to enter the thought processes of another species, she turned to look at—or more properly to listen to—the minds of others via psychoanalysis, leaving objective detachment behind. The irony for my present purpose is that Freud wanted to picture others' inner motives and states by listening and never by looking at the face.

Though for that reason I left Freud behind, I did learn from psychoanalysis the importance of individuals' stories and the need to enter into their experience; external objective observation seemed insufficient for my purpose. But if not a displayer of signals and behaviors as in animals, what then does the face do? It is the window of the soul, of course, allowing insight into the thoughts and motives of others. How this might have developed I discuss next, in chapter 6, contrasting the views of cognitive psychology and psychotherapy. These ideas about "theories of mind," or how we know of other people's minds and feelings, are embedded—or made flesh—by exploring the problems which autistic subjects have with the faces of other people.

People with autism and Asperger syndrome have multiple problems in sensory processing, social interaction, language and communication, and cognition itself. They have also been said to ignore the faces of other people. I show rather that autistic subjects actively *avoid* the face, to avoid complex signals of mood in other people, which on the one hand they can hardly decipher, and on the other threaten to overwhelm them. This is taken further, in chapter 7, in an interview with Donna Williams, an autistic savant who has explored her condition and its effects on her relations and interactions with others in an unique and very moving way. What she can and cannot take from the face of others reveals something of what autism is, and much about our own experience of the face as well.

Autism is not just about facial expression, of course. There is, however, a condition, Möbius syndrome, in which people are born without any ability to move their faces and so cannot make facial expressions. In chapters 8 and 9 their experiences are set against experimental work on the importance of the face and facial expression in the development of social skills and interactions in children. The stories of those with Möbius allow some understanding of what it is like to grow up without facial movement and the effect that has not only on one's social existence, but on how the immobility of the face affects the experience of emotion itself.

There may be large differences in the experiences of those born without facial mobility and those in whom it occurs later which tell indirectly of the problems in development without facial mobility. In chapter 10 I explore the experiences of those who have lost facial expression as adults and who are often considered to have become dull and boring. Fortunately, there are ways of helping such people, and with renewed facial animation often comes renewed enthusiasm for life. One such program is detailed that has proved useful to people with Parkinson's disease.

Lastly, I went to see people with facial disfigurements. Recently, an organization in the United Kingdom, Changing Faces, has been helping and encouraging those with disfigurements. Often their clients are so ashamed of themselves—their facial selves—that they have become socially isolated, reclusive, and devoid of self-esteem. One of their first tasks is to look at themselves and then to gain the courage simply to look at someone else, since to look and so invite mutual gaze requires a reciprocity and relationship.

The heart of this book, then, resides in the experiences of people with facial losses of various forms. In their loss of function is revealed something of what all our faces reflect. These biographical accounts are used, together with scientific data, to develop ideas about the role of the evolution of the face in the development of social interaction, social intelligence, and human development.

A highly developed face is unique to our species. In animals there is a gradual movement from the display and prediction of behavior to the expression of inner states in higher primates and man. The development of the face has, therefore, taken place in parallel with the evolution of these complex inner states themselves. Indeed, a mobile expressive face may have been crucial for this intellectual development. One reason for the success of primates has been their development of complex social groups. These require regulation, based on mutual regard and hierarchy, and I suggest that facial display has a role in this. In humans further advances have occurred which enable, through mutual regard, ways into others' minds.

This mind reading should not be thought of as being concerned about cognition alone, in terms of reading thoughts and predicting actions. I suggest that this ability to look into another's mind may have begun in an affective, feeling domain. Intelligence itself may have arisen socially to regulate complex social groups, rather than as a way of storing knowledge of the external world. If social intelligence was required for the development of an understanding of others' feelings, then it is difficult to imagine its development without some external discloser of those feeling states. I suggest a crucial role for the face in this, though other channels like vocalization and body posture cannot be excluded. These matters may not be of evolutionary significance alone. Babies and children first reach out to the world not via abstract thoughts but through a relatedness to others based on an affective emotional need, and much of this relatedness is communicated through facial expression. If this is the case, then the face has a role in the child's development of socialization and in the realization of others.[3]

In the final chapter I bring together the disparate clinical conditions of blindness, autism, Möbius syndrome, Parkinson's disease, and facial disfigurement to show the relations between them and how they all allow us to know something of how we are defined by our faces. From scientific evidence I advance a natural history of the face, postulating for it a role in the development of consciousness. In parallel, I discuss the importance of facial embodiment for our well-being and suggest how that well-being depends on an emotional sensibility revealed to others via the face. This development has ended at, or at least has thus far reached, levels of cognitive thought and abstraction beyond that which the face can disclose through the development of language. I end, however, by emphasizing the importance of the emotional and social aspects of our being and how they are linked through an embodiment in which facial action plays an essential part.

"Tell, Please"

But these ideas came after I had first been moved by Mary's case. After the case conference I finished my work and then went to the ward, introduced myself to Mary, and sat with her. Her family came and through her daughter Kate, slowly, her story emerged.

Eight years before I met them Kate had thought her mother's speech sounded a little slurred on the phone. But the change was slow and she took little notice. Mary herself blamed her husband George for not listening, and thought he was going deaf. She even sent him off to an audiologist to have his ears tested. Two years later they moved to be nearer their daughter in Hampshire, by which the time her speech had worsened. Mother and daughter had always enjoyed each other's company and enjoyed a laugh, so they laughed about this too. Kate remembers from about this time that if her parents came for a meal her mother would eat very little. Mary would say that she did not feel hungry, or that she had eaten too much at home. But even when at her mother's, Kate noticed that Mary ate little; slowly, she began to lose weight.

Kate would go around to visit her. If the TV was on, then Mary would just appear to look at it, occasionally saying a few words to her daughter, but there would be none, could be none, of the fast flow of facial expression and words that conversation implies. They used to talk and gossip nonstop, and now there was no interplay of words or facial expressions. Kate missed her mother enormously, for it was as if she had gone.

Her mother went from 168 pounds down to 126 pounds and Kate was concerned, but Mary made light of it and so nothing was done. Eventually Kate made her mother go to see Dr. Fawkes at the local hospital. Kate did most of the talking, difficult because much had been hidden from her by Mary and George, and she had no idea how bad her mother had become at home. By then Mary's speech was nearly nonexistent and she had taken to writing most things down. She had acquired a Lightwriter, a small portable typewriter, from a service for disabled people, and had almost given up speech altogether. Dr. Fawkes asked how long ago Mary had lost her facial expression, and up to that time Kate had not realized it had gone. No one had. They had all put it down to her sadness about the illness and had thought she had lost her sense of humor. Even George was unaware of it.

When Dr. Fawkes admitted her to hospital it really hit Kate. She and George had to answer the questions; Mary was put in a side room with no TV. She just sat there, unable to communicate except through her Lightwriter. She occasionally walked around the wards but neither the nurses nor the other patients knew quite how to deal with her. She could hardly speak, or move her face, and few people had the time or the inclination to sit down and wait for her to tap out "Hello, how are you?" on the machine.

Tests did not reveal any cause for the problem (they had feared cancer). She was fitted with a small stomach tube for liquid nourishment. Once home she cooked for George but could not eat herself. George became embarrassed to eat and enjoy food in front of her and so he took to eating in another room. She became depressed, though the only facial expression she could manage was when the tears trickled down her impassive cheeks.

Before her illness she had been a very active member of the local Women's Institute. It had been hard for her to sit through an evening meeting after she fell ill, because she would often cough. She also felt that people talked as though she were not there, or as if she were stupid. She was a very gifted flower arranger, and when she was strong enough she offered to do an evening's demonstration. Since she could not talk her way through the actions she had spent hours writing down the commentary for her daughter. Kate, however, told her mother that she was too shy to read them out and got someone else to do it. In fact, Kate was so affected by her mother's courage that she could not have done it. Mary cried at the end when they applauded. But she could not take questions or give any advice and soon afterward she left the group.

Kate would go around and have a laugh with her mother as usual, except that something was missing: the inevitable disagreements and playful squabblings between mother and daughter. Her mother's emotional highs and lows were no longer there. Kate just put it down to her mother's concern about her illness.

Slowly, despite the stomach tube and the devoted help of Kate and George, Mary got thinner and more disabled. She had always used the expression "going home" as a euphemism for dying. One day she tapped out that she would like to go home to see the village in which she had grown up. They all had a day trip and she saw the cottage she was born in. The lady owner invited her in and showed her around. A lovely respite from her illness, but from then on when she tapped "going home" it could only mean one thing. She began to fall at home. Kate once picked her up and asked playfully what on earth they could do with her. Mary just tapped out "going home."

I went to visit her on a few occasions. Conversation was slow, because of the typewriter, but I soon felt at ease with her pace, waiting for the words and small sentences. Sitting with her one afternoon she typed, "fed up," and then "lonely."

"But George looks after you." A little later, "Benji want out."

George lets the dog out. There is a box of tissues next to her chair; she salivates constantly and can just manage to wipe the saliva away from the slack unmoving mouth she is left with. "I can't cough."

When she tries to cough her eyes do wrinkle a little more but there is no movement in the mouth or lower face. The forehead also twitches a little, but so little that you have to watch for that and nothing else. There is little remaining of the normal, whole, live, animated movement of the face we take for granted. Sitting with her conversing slowly, in her new time, the lack of facial movement seemed to imprison and threaten her sense of self. Fed, after a fashion, and comfortably looked after, what was missing was an engagement with others, even with her family, which seemed to have gone with her loss of facial animation. I asked what she enjoyed.

"Jane."

Her friend comes in once a week while George goes out to do the shopping. They converse "on machine." No one else comes in except Kate, of course. No one from the Women's Institute. As if reading my thoughts she tapped out, "I can't alter my expression."

She had many things wrong. The swallowing difficulty made eating and drinking virtually impossible. These were major problems, but were, in a way, private to her. The loss of speech had prevented gossip, but she heard the news from Kate and from her friends. It was her loss of facial expressiveness, which had initially not even been noticed, that was an important reason for her feeling so distant, and that had contributed so much to her loss of friends and companions. Without the ability to relate to people through, and with, the face, she was reduced in their and her eyes as a person, as a being, *as her*.

Though conversation was possible, few people found the time. For without the feedback and reinforcement between people that facial gestures provide, there was little relatedness and engagement. Her loss of facial responsiveness made her feel somehow invalidated at her very core.

She blinks, there is a small eye wrinkle and a chesty noise. No laugh. but there is almost a grimace on her face.

"I laugh Benji. Would you make cup?"

She orders George about. We laugh and she joins in as best she can. He says that the last time I was there she had so much to say but not enough time; her writing was so slow on the machine. She has so much to say,

"I find I think very well as us no." A pause. "I think as well as before. No tea."

She has got George to make me some, but does not want any herself. She writes slowly and is maddened if people end her sentences for her. She is maddened if people assume she has any intellectual loss, a common assumption since they think her loss of facial reaction reflects a dementia. She hates interruptions, so I sit and listen, sit and watch. The pace is slow but soon becomes imperceptible, irrelevant. The Lightwriter is a lifeline.

"I use the machine. Thanks for seeing me."

It is my pleasure. I ask if I might someday write something about her story. If she agrees.

"Write. Tell, please."

She died two months later after a further stroke, then pneumonia. She had for years tapped out to her daughter, "Come and see me." Kate knew it was not what it meant—for she visited every day. It was Mary asking for her to check that she looked all right once she was dead. After a further stroke she tapped to Kate, "I wish I were dead." There had been no trivia, no gossip for years and yet the starkness of this made Kate struggle hard to hold her tears. She had no reply, just a hug.

She went into the hospital. A pleasant enough ward, but there was no one with the time or the understanding to look at the Lightwriter. No one came to look after her, for she could give nothing in return. During this time Kate's half-sister, Liz, who had not visited for years, phoned. When Kate went in to see her mother Mary wrote "love you," on the writer. She did it several times, and then used the repeat button, "love you," "love you," "love you," Kate thought that her mother was passing on a message from her long-lost sister. It took her a long time to realize that her mother was not referring to Liz's call, but was expressing her love for Kate, again and again in the only way she could, tapping out letters on a screen.

The next Monday Kate could not visit, the only day she did not go. That was the day Mary died. Afterward Kate did go and see her, and she looked more like her mother, more at peace. In death she had an expression that had been beyond her in life.

Looking through the Window

Mary had lost the ability to swallow and to talk and she had little movement in her limbs.[4] So surely her facial problem was trivial compared with these other matters? And yet sitting with her I reached another conclusion. Her lack of self-expressiveness, and resulting social isolation, was an almost unimaginable loss, a loss so profound that she was overwhelmed by it as much as by the other problems. It was so profound that she was concerned for her facial expression even in death. The face, *her* face, was somehow more part of her self, *her* soul, than the swallowing or the weak arm.

If the face or the eyes are the window of the soul, then this well-known metaphor is more apt than is usually realized. When she first lost facial expression no one noticed—they just assumed she was depressed or fed up. Just as the deaf were considered stupid because they lacked language, so she became less of an individual, less of a person, because she could not show her animated self. Rather than seeing the face for what it was, everyone looked straight through the window and saw her mood and personality, or so they thought.

Though by my training I am academic in approach, sitting with Mary I began to realize the importance of delving into the experience of individuals with unusual facial problems. Only they had been forced deep into the experience of the face that had interested me, and moved me, from the start. So I went next to talk with several blind people, reasoning that if the face had significance for the congenitally blind, then it would reflect on how deep the concept of faces might be within us. While outwardly similar to the congenitally blind, those with late onset-blindness turned out to inhabit a very different world, having constructed it—and their perception of themselves and their loved ones—visually. What might it mean to *lose* sight of one's family and one's self, and what part of that loss was a facial loss? I begin therefore with the experiences of four blind people. In searching for how the face defines our existence, by looking at the consequences of facial loss, they seemed the place to start.

Residing in Voices

The face evolved to be seen by others. We build up ideas of ourselves and others which are predominantly visual in nature. When asked to think of someone, we picture the person and picture particularly his or her face. How, then, do those who have never seen build up character? I went to talk with people blind from birth.

One might think that sighted people can imagine what it is like to be blind. After all, it is easy to close your eyes. But wait a moment; this is a colossal oversimplification, for when sighted people close their eyes they still *imagine* the world in visual terms. They still know their way around a room or know what their loved ones look like. Vision still dominates not only our view of the world but our concepts of person, for our perception of people is encompassed to a large extent by what they look like, and particularly by what their faces look like.

"Not Like a Hand"

Peter White is in his forties and works for the BBC as a radio and television journalist. He went blind as a young baby and has no recollection of seeing anything but ill-defined shades of light. He has presented *In Touch,* a radio program for visually handicapped people in Britain, for many years. Many sighted listeners are also drawn to the program because of the warmth and friendliness of Peter's voice. More recently he has fulfilled an ambition to work in mainstream television as a feature presenter. I sat with Peter over a BBC lunch. I asked if he had ever considered what he might be missing in seeing the faces of others, with all the expressions and individuality they communicated.

"I've never thought about that before. I think I contain most of myself in my voice. That's where I reside. If you ask me what conveys most externally about who I am, I would say my voice. Partly in what I say but very much in tones and how I say it."

"But are there differences between what can be said, which is often factual, and the emotional, affective aspect of communication, which may not be fully in the voice? Is that where facial expression is important, or can the voice contain these nuances?"

He replied obliquely, and from his own experience. "I'm very aware of my wife's moods—aren't we all? I can talk to her on the phone and I say 'What's wrong?' She is annoyed because she is such a giveaway. All right, so there must be other people who are less open about their moods, or that I'm less concerned about to pick up moods in, or people I just don't care about."

This suggested that blindness may impose an intimacy, a level of knowledge applied only to those people known well. A sighted person has knowledge of many people at many levels of acquaintance. Perhaps blind people can know about a relatively few people at a certain level of intimacy, suggesting that facial expression may have more universals of expression than the voice. All the more remarkable then that Peter spends his life interviewing people he has never met.

I asked Peter if he could find in the voice emotions that for sighted people might be seen in the face.

"Yes, certainly. It is not only in the voice, there are also different qualities of silence. A contented silence when you know that she's just been talking to you and that she is doing something else, and a silence when you know she's quiet because if she said something it would be absolutely appalling."

"It is still difficult to imagine that all the moods and expressions which pass across the face rapidly, like clouds' shadows across a field, have a similar representation in the voice. As an outsider I would be concerned that the emotional range which the voice conveys is different and slightly more limited than that conveyed by facial expression."

"It's very hard for me to know. All that I do know is that, on the whole, my track record within the family or among friends can be quicker and more accurate than my wife's. There are nuances in conversation. For instance, I will say to her 'Didn't you think that so-and-so meant such-and-such?' and she'll say 'Oh, I didn't notice.' More times than not I will be right. I wouldn't for a minute think that the voice and the face are conveying the same thing but they may well be conveying aspects of the same thing."

"Are you aware at some level of the expressiveness of the face, of your face?"

"Yes, of course, my expressiveness is in the mouth, isn't it?"

Looking and talking with Peter one soon is oblivious to his blindness. His whole face is animated, interested, immersed in the conversation. I try, feebly, to suggest as much.

"Maybe that's why people haven't balked at putting me on television. My wife says I have a very expressive face that looks very engaged. I get very bold with people so that when I am arguing with someone I lean forward, bringing my face toward them. That's how I feel."

We are both leaning over the table now as we become involved. "Is there," I ask, "a need to present one's face to the person one is engaged with?"

"The face is not doing something that's very conscious. It's not doing something that's vital to my existence, but it is doing something that I want to communicate. You are aware at some level that in order to interact and talk with people you present your face to them. It's not just a place where your voice comes out of. I think it's possibly a reflection of wanting to make contact with them."

"May I return to an earlier question? Are there certain feelings which are heard more in the voice, as others are seen better on the face?"

"I think I would happily concede that. I have always been fairly conscious of the smile. A smile is a physical entity to a blind person because of the sensation that it generates inside yourself. Its almost in the throat, a bubbly feeling. You're not necessarily going to laugh. You can feel your face twist and certain muscles relax so you know intellectually that this changes the shape of your face."

"One may, however, perhaps experience some increased accuracy and some feedback of mood from the expression of your face. And this refinement may not be the same in the blind."

"I admit that you may. Oddly enough, doing my job the thing people say most about me is that I have a smile in my voice. I wonder if I put it there rather than putting it on my face as a conscious or non-conscious way of communicating positive feedback to other people.

"One of the things about being blind is the amount of help you need, and one of the things which is very clear is that people receive help if they look open. I suspect that facial expression is a big indicator of that. I know blind people who complain that they don't get help and it's my suspicion that they don't look as though they want it.

"I don't know how much I give away of myself in sadness. I am aware of noncommunication, of my face tightening up and closing up. You would have to ask someone else about how much my face reveals when I am sad because I am not necessarily so aware of it as in smiling. Maybe sighted people aren't either."

"Smiling and laughing are loud in a way in which most sadness is not. We very rarely make noises when we are sad or distraught, but are often noisy when happy. Is it possible, therefore, that perception of emotional range by blind people in others differs?"

"I think I put a smile on my face when I consciously want to be helped, and I know how to put a smile on my face. I don't know which comes first, whether I was happily, luckily, equipped with a smile, or whether I've decided you get the best results in getting what you want if you do smile."

Darwin used the fact that congenitally blind children develop facial expression normally as evidence for its innateness.[1] Peter's expressions are, to all appearances, normal. I returned to him. "Do you know when someone is speaking to you if they're looking at you, and do you reciprocate?"

"Yes. It's to say I'm interested in you. It's you I'm directing this at. I don't think anyone taught me to do this. Your head is not only where your smile comes from. It seems natural to point it in the right direction toward someone."

"May I ask an inevitable question, though by now I have an idea of the answer. Does blindness leave you free from some of the distractions of the world?"

"I don't like the idea that sees compensations in blindness. If you can hear the voice and you can see the face you've got two sources of evidence, and two's better than one. I grew up needing to fill time so that I did not have to think intensely all the time. It always amuses me when people say blind people make such good employees because they're not distracted. I always think, 'Bollocks'—I'm distracted by all sorts of things: other people, people to talk to, half-heard jokes across a crowded room. My brain is doing its damnedest the whole time to distract me and I wonder if that's not a function of, or a reaction of, someone who's lost their sight early. If all that visual information left a gap, I filled that gap in when I was a kid.[2] I wanted to be distracted with sounds. I love jokes, I love eavesdropping and voices. I can't turn my ears off, no, but I can turn the signals off a bit. I can become absorbed in sounds as much as anyone, and just as I can be absorbed in a book in Braille."

Lunch was over; in fact, we were the only ones left in the canteen. Peter made his way back to prepare for the evening TV news program, or maybe for a talk show on local radio, or another edition of the program for blind listeners. Whichever it was, he set off with relish and optimism, ready to discuss and debate with another interviewee.

Peter had first gained success as a radio interviewer in a medium perhaps suited to blind people. Next I went to talk with a man whose whole professional life had been very much in the sighted world, in the rough and tumble of national politics.

A Politician Who Finds It Difficult to Smile

David Blunkett is MP for Sheffield Brightside and now Secretary of State for Education and Employment, a key appointment in Prime Minister Tony Blair's new Labour Government. Before his education brief he was shadow Secretary of State for Health. He has also been blind since birth. I began by apologizing for coming to talk to him about the effect of his disability rather than about his ability. He did not mind at all. I began with a famous adversary of his, and most of his party.

"If someone said 'What's Margaret Thatcher like?' I would describe her. Mitterand said she had the lips of Monroe and a smile like Caligula. I would describe physical visible features."

"My picture is, in my view, entirely different to likely physical makeup—but I am influenced by what people tell me. So I know Neil Kinnock [ex-leader of the Labour Party] has gone bald and that he started to wear funereal suits. I know this from listening to people and compiling a picture. It's very hard to describe how someone can see a visual picture when they cannot physically see the person, but it is possible. I can envisage a person, but not in detail, not their nose, not their eyes, just the person, and build it up.

"I will get a picture from someone's voice. Margaret Thatcher was a classic example who was by nature stern: I can imagine the flash in the eyes and the face, a glare. Incidentally I have to be very careful not to glare when I don't intend to glare. You don't smile when you don't want to smile, unless you're a good actor, but it is possible to look stern and to glare when you don't actually mean to. I have to control my voice also; I can be very sharp when I don't mean to be. If I upset with a voice, then I'm even more likely to upset with a look of disdain or boredom, which I don't feel but I may have just drifted off for a minute."

He is obviously aware of the face disclosing feelings and mood. As a corollary to this he seems aware also of the need to control it, when the nonverbal feedback from others to alert him to the effect his facial expression is having on others is absent. But he is almost describing another thing. By residing in the voice and not to the same extent in the face, his face may not be so accurately reflecting his feelings, and yet, being seen by others, allows misinterpretations which he is poorly aware of. He seems to need to be vigilant about this.

"On television I have to remember that people are more impressed, or depressed, by how you look than by what you say. I find that very hard work and have to concentrate. Politics is now so much image and atmosphere, and I have to remember that.

"When I was much younger, when I first came into politics, my first television interview was very difficult. My eyes flick and move around, not desperately and it doesn't matter, but it did matter to several viewers. Some people, who didn't know that I couldn't see, wrote to say that I looked devious because I wasn't looking straight into the camera. A fellow interviewee suggested dark glasses but I said 'No way, I'm not going to wear dark glasses, I'm going to be me and if people don't understand, then they must learn to.' I asked another interviewer to introduce me as 'David Blunkett with his guide dog, Ruby.' I don't have to do that any more because people tend to know me. Rather than being a blind person and hiding behind dark glasses it was necessary to find a little way round it for my own psychological confidence.

"Facial expression is very important in the House of Commons. Logically the members know that I can't see them. But if they pass me in the corridor and I don't acknowledge them their intelligence tells them I can't see, therefore don't take offence, but their instincts override it. I know they do because people have actually indicated that to me on more than one occasion."

"Charles Bell said that, 'the thought is to the word as the feeling is to the facial expression.'"[3]

"And I have to remember that. People expect that. I have to keep trying. I should express myself verbally and with touch far more. I also have to remember—and this is the other side of the coin—not to verbalize everything. Good friends at home have said, 'Don't babble on,' as compared with the alternative, which would be just looking. I'm not worried by silence per se as long as I know the context in which it has arisen. So if I had a row with one of my boys then I would want to know if they'd gone or not, but otherwise I usually know why the silence has occurred."

"Alain Prost, the Grand Prix driver, said that he was fed up with motor racing because it was just like politics—it was trying to get people to believe things about driving abilities, speed of car, use of tires, and so forth, with less regard for the facts. Much of this hidden agenda is expressed not through words but through various other forms of expression, both in facial expression and body language."

"People have said to me recently that part of the difficulty fellow politicians in the House of Commons have in relating to you is that sometimes your body language is very dismissive. Now, there's a thought. Does that mean my face is dismissive? Am I dismissive in my manner, face, and other actions, and do I have to think about that and at my time of life? I'm forty-seven. It's interesting to have to think about that."

Again he seemed to be considering a dissociation between the thought, the feeling, and his facial expression. I thought of how awful to be in a place like the Commons and have that leveled at you, something so important and yet so out of one's own control. Blindness is perhaps unique in its asymmetry—the blind are always on show to the world and yet unable to receive any such signals about others, or gain much feedback about the effect of their appearance on others. I returned to David.

"Peter White has his beautiful friendly voice and he's aware, as a communicator, that he has to put people at their ease, though as he said he thinks the smile in his voice is always there. Do you think that your lack of sight has imposed on you a certain austerity?"

"Yes, my friends say that the problem on television is that I look far too serious. 'For God's sake,' they say, 'don't do a sickly smile,' which I couldn't do anyway. 'Just try and smile a bit.' They ask me to just remember that people viewing don't always want to see me reflecting the austerity of the thoughts I may be having inside. Now, there's an interesting idea. It is very difficult because I am concentrating extremely hard on the question and on my answer and I'm forgetting about facial expression. You forget that automatically people are viewing you, and as you've grown up without that you have to think of it and superimpose some facial reaction onto the rest of your thoughts."

"But when you're out gossiping with your friends it all just happens. Are you suggesting that it is more difficult to do it in a public arena?"

"Yes. I'm a politician who finds it difficult to smile on cue, though not all politicians find this. [I had learned by now to detect David's comic understatements.] I rejoice in radio."

I had the impression that he had had so much political success by sheer hard work, with little awareness by his colleagues of just how difficult it was. "There is also a reluctance of people in my own party to address these things with me. They are so frightened of raising it that they miss the point. I don't mind addressing these issues at all, that's why I'm talking to you, but they don't know that so they move round it. For instance, I have been a member of the shadow cabinet for over two years and I've held the health brief and now the education one. They have never asked me to take part in a party political broadcast. I wonder in the back of my mind if they are worried about my presentation and visual skills."

I could see the party fixers' problem, but thought them wrong, for David was probably the most famous blind person in England, but more than that, people knew him as the Labour politician who was blind, and not the other way round. "Sighted people feel that they reside in their face. Peter White said that his characterization of people resides in the voice."

"If I am honest the voice is very important but I also weigh other people's views, though I never take a single person's viewpoint. I find that people with very pleasant voices, though not exclusively, generally have pleasant faces. Not necessarily beautiful, but pleasant and attractive. Now that's very sad for people with attractive voices or an attractive face but not both. It may be that the person with the rough voice may be wonderful. Fortunately, we all see different things, both in our perceptions and our voice and in our visual appreciation of them. Otherwise the world would be a terrible place, because some people would be excluded for no good reason.

"It is very important we understand that, and that's important for people's perceptions of facial expression. Some of us [the blind] can't see and appreciate the importance of our face and manner and body language for other people. We therefore do not think about it. We ought to learn about it at school. Blind children smile when they are happy or enjoying something, but they do not naturally do a social smile, when it is expected, and that has to be suggested to them. It should be part of our social development, which it isn't, certainly wasn't in my day. Secondly, we should learn a little about other people's expressions and even learn, because you *can* learn how to do this, how someone's change of voice indicates a change of facial expression and a change of mood. It's very important to try and integrate blind people into the world of the sighted. One way is to try and introduce them to the social aspects and I accept that, for most people, 'social' means facial expression.

"I'm halfway through my life, and I need to start anew. I still pick up nuances from voices but I am still not sure, absolutely sure, that I've got down to a fine art the twinkle in the eye from the voice. I pick up other things, for instance, coughing when I'm speaking at a meeting when I've lost the audience, but it's not infallible. I have not fully understood the really intimate smile and I am working on it."

"That must be magnified in the Commons when you miss a lot because you can only hear it."

"Yes, of course, and then there's no alternative, I just have to ask. I am also desperately developing other ways of picking things up. I use my imagination when I watch a film, for instance. I just put two and two together and may make five, but sometimes a plot I've developed is better than the original. The other thing to remember is that it is not just the visual set of your face—when you're delivering an irony or a joke you have to do a look so people have got the idea visually of what you're trying to transfer. I am not a great hands-all-over-the-place person, but it is useful sometimes to indicate visually what you're getting across verbally. I do sometimes forget that and I can appear wooden because of it."

"Returning to my comment about austerity—you're not aware of having such good body or facial vocabulary to set beside your vocal one?"

"That's right, I think you're right. Austere is a good word and it can be misinterpreted, given the sensitivity of politicians, which is unmatched anywhere else I should think except in the theatre."

"Because you're performing and your advancement and self-esteem depend on others, and their perception of you depends on what you look like and how you act."

"Yes, it's interesting. What's very important for blind persons is they mustn't become introverted or paranoid. There are lessons to be learned and things to be done with youngsters but it's then best just to relax and live."

At this point Big Ben chimed the hour and David was due in committee. He made his apologies and reminded me that I had arranged to interview his staff. I left the House of Commons and walked through the sunshine to his offices overlooking the river. His secretaries told me how they could go for several days without seeing him. They said that it seemed to make little difference to David whether he was talking on the telephone or face to face. Otherwise there was little they could say. David, they said, was just David—his blindness was irrelevant to the way they considered him.

It was similar when I spoke with Peter White's wife and son. Peter was Peter, considered just like anyone else, his lack of sight irrelevant to their perception of him as a person. They could not step back to focus on his use of facial expression, for that they accepted as part of the whole, part of *his* whole. For the blind, as for any "disabled" person, the disability becomes less relevant to those who know them well. It is more of a stigma for those who do not know the person, when first, often superficial, impressions assume more importance (see chapter 11).

David Blunkett can't go into lobbies or tearooms and smile and greet people normally as politicians do because he doesn't know who's there. He has to wait for people to come to him, producing a distance which is very difficult in politics. He finds two particular problems: the amount of sheer work he has to listen to in order to keep up, and his difficulties in the socializing which is such an essential part of politics. To be the only blind MP among 659 must be enormously distancing. It must be much more difficult to try to learn six hundred to a thousand voices than it is to remember that number of faces and voices, for we learn faces effortlessly. In *Immortality* Milan Kundera wrote, "You know me by my face, you know me as a face, and you never knew me in any other way. Therefore it could not occur to you that my face is not my self."[4]

Knowing no other existence, Peter's and David's minds and worlds were filled by sound. Their experience of others, and of their character and mood, are from voice and through their auditory imagination. One might even say that these two blind persons had constituted the "face" of others differently. For them the other's "face," meaning the person's representation of character, mood, and even perhaps self, was not encompassed by his or her physical face or visual appearance but almost by a "virtual face"—a representation of another's individuality constituted in voice.[5] Yet from both I got the sense that the physical face remained important, as a means of communication and as a way of initiating and controlling personal attention, and so of reaching out to others.

I had floated the idea that facial expression and voice may communicate slightly different aspects of emotional information. In fact, there is some work differentiating this. Klaus Scherer has suggested that facial expression may convey the pleasant or unpleasant elements of a person's mood, whereas the voice is better at revealing the level of arousal, from terror at one end of the spectrum to contentment at the other. Despite this, emotional recognition is obviously possible from voice; for instance, sadness is slow and relatively monotonous. Vivien Tartter has provided evidence of how normal listeners can tell "happy talk," when the speaker is smiling, from the voice.[6] Talking with Peter and David, however, both blind from birth, I had the impression that though there might be some differences in their abilities in these matters, they had learned to compensate. The situation might, however, be very different in someone who went blind as a adult.

I had talked to two exceptional people, whose worlds were crammed full of words and details and activity. They had never known any other life. As I left him, David turned and said, "There are very few downsides to living without sight simply because you've always lived without it. But of course it's a very different matter if you have lost your sight." I wanted to know how it was different. How did those who go blind as adults move from a dependence on visual communication between themselves and others, and a social existence with vision, to a life in which they know they will never be able to see again? Such people would be in a position to reflect on these differences in experience in a manner those blind from birth could not.

We Do Not Share the Same World

3

For those blind from birth, as we have seen, it is clear that voice is the source of personal identification and character. For Peter White voice is all—a seamless, adequate channel for communication and feelings. But what of those who became blind as adults? Their whole view of the world and their imagination would have been visual. How might they experience loss of sight and, in particular, the loss of the sight of the faces of others and of themselves? I explored these issues with two people who had become blind as adults, one two years after the event, another over ten years later.

Floods of Faces

Until the age of twenty-one Jeremy could see clearly, but by twenty-three, despite several operations, he could see nothing. For the first year he felt surprisingly strong despite the daily inconveniences, but then, slowly, he found life becoming more and more difficult. Initially, when meeting new people and making new friends, he could not put a face to them, so he began by explaining his problem and asking to feel people's faces. To his despair he soon found it impossible to construct a face in the mind from feeling it with his hands. Knowing the particularity of each person's face he was moved to write that he had wished he had never seen. The lucky ones had been blind since birth.

It was apparent when I met Jeremy that whereas Peter White had never had visual imagery, Jeremy's own inner life was awash with it, and that at times he was scarcely able to control it. On the underground, going to and from work, a face would appear in his mind and take over all other thoughts. It might be the face of a loved one, or the face of a child from earlier school years whom he had not seen for years, but who still filled his mind. He would not see a vague face, as if there were such things, but an actual one. Though in the year or so since going blind all sorts of visual memories had flooded his consciousness, the memory of faces had been the most important of all. These faces of children from his schooldays, whom he had not seen for years, appeared in a scarcely controllable manner. Those faces, which he scarcely remembered when sighted, crowded his imagination, upsetting and disquieting him with their insistence and because he knew that he would never see them again.

He was caught between a desire to hold onto a visual world, even with visual imagery he could not control, and the thought that this existence would never be replenished and so would always be rooted in the past. Being blind meant that he could only look back, in an internal, unshared, world. The more imagery of face that he could keep, then the greater his hold on the world and the greater sense he could make of it. Listening to Jeremy it seemed that for him to go blind was to lose some of his bearings not just of the geographic world but also of the connections with others that face and gaze and eye contact previously, imperceptibly, had provided.

While as a sighted person he found it very difficult to remember faces, once blind, paradoxically, it was easier, and the faces that he remembered were more precious and he strove to hang onto them, hanging onto the love and friendships they represented and embodied. He played games with new people. Unable to construct their faces, he invented new ones for them. He would think of people they reminded him of, and then used those persons' faces for the new person. This made it easier for him to get on with those persons, though there was trouble when people behaved in a different way from those whose faces he had given them. This creative use of visual memory to sustain and enrich new friendships was neat and clever, but it was necessarily backward looking. He was aware of this and also found that it could not be sustained.

He felt strong for the first couple of years after going blind, but then slowly his confidence drained away. His depression at this time corresponded with the time that this precious visual imagery began to fade. In a sense his leaving of the visual world had been not when he became blind but when his visual memory was no longer clear, and this was when he found himself at his lowest. Without vision he also lost much of the affective or feeling quality associated with it and had been unable to regain or transfer this through other channels. No more sights of sunny days or pretty girls, no longer would food look good, no more colors to brighten his day. But most of all no more faces and facial expressions, no more stolen glances or cheeky grins, no more conversations through looking: this loss defined his isolation. Trying to cheer him up, friends said that for him some people would stay forever young. In the course of his work he had recently met an actress, a ex-star of British films he remembers as a nubile and voluptuous young woman in her early twenties. He was thrilled to meet her and they became friends. He treats her as a young woman, and naturally she adores this, for she is now eighty.

Fortunately, after a period of depression, Jeremy began to explore the relationship between voice and mood without the comfort of facial expression. Where Peter White "filled the gap," unconsciously and effortlessly as a child, Jeremy began to realize the problems inherent in "just" talking to people. If they suddenly go quiet, for instance, he is completely unaware of what they are thinking or doing. He does not know if they are reflective, or having a wry laugh. He is in a no man's land waiting for another sound, for a context to rejoin the conversation.

It was apparent that two or three years after going blind he was beginning to make himself available to other ways of knowing about the world and about others. He had just got back from a weekend in the country and had enjoyed its sounds and smells and the wholeness of its experience. We finished our meal and I took Jeremy by the arm and dropped him off at his girlfriend's house. Out in the street he mentioned that he was a keen musician. He plays every day, works from memory, and performs in public a few times a year. And when playing the violin he is no longer conscious of being blind.

Sweating Blood

John Hull is Professor of Religious Education and Dean of the Faculty of Education and Continuing Studies at the University of Birmingham. He has been writing articles and books on biblical exegesis and theology for years to the general approval of colleagues. But his book, *Touching the Rock,* published in 1990, led to a wholly different level of interest. It gave an astonishing account of his experience during the first few years following the loss of his sight.[1] It exposed the crudity and lack of imagination with which most of us sighted people approach the world of the blind.

Born in North East Victoria, Australia, John first noticed difficulty in seeing when he was thirteen. Cataract was diagnosed and soon after that he lost sight in the right eye. A few months later the same process began in the left eye. He had several successful operations to dissolve the cataracts, though at the price of wearing thick glasses. Then four or five years later he noticed a dark disk-shaped area in his visual field. It was the beginning of a far more serious problem: retinal detachment. Fortunately several operations led to good return of function. Successful at school, he went onto Cambridge to study theology. He absorbed all that Cambridge could give, and spent his spare time on a motor scooter traveling around England and hitchhiking around Europe and the Middle East. He became a teacher in London before reaching Birmingham, initially as a lecturer in divinity. It was two years after this that the shadow reappeared. By 1973, despite expert medical care, he was using a magnifying glass to read; in 1977 he knew he had read his last novel. For the next three years he could just about read for work, but by 1980, at the age of forty-five, he knew that the detachments could no longer be fought or ignored as they had been for thirty years. Three years later the last light sensations faded and with that he began, finally, to disclose his feelings in the diary that became his book.

In his diary John described many of the same experiences as Jeremy, though John's account covered a much longer period. There was, for instance, a time when images of faces appeared so strongly that they were almost uncontrollable, like hallucinations. Listening to people, vivid pictures would pop up, like looking at a TV set, and would so engross him that he would lose the thread of conversation. In the hospital, when he had been temporarily without sight, he would construct images of what people looked like, only to have them shattered when the bandages came off and he could see. He described how in the first few years of blindness people fell into two groups: those with faces and those without. It was a bit like wandering around the National Portrait Gallery with rows of portraits and every so often a gap on the wall. He could tell where the portrait used to be because of the outline on the wallpaper. He found that the people he had met before going blind had faces but those since blindness did not, and he found it very difficult to relate the two groups to each other. As time passed the gallery became barer. In the first three years of blindness the pictures of those he had known before but had not encountered during that time were still on the wall, but those of the people he met everyday were not. He was replacing their visual iconic memory with something more dependent on his continued experience of them.

Most distressing was that he was beginning to forget what his wife and children looked like. He had sworn to himself that he would carry their faces forever, even if everything else in the gallery was stolen. He tried to hold onto these by imagining a photograph, a static image with a border. But however much he tried, even these images faded. He also lost a knowledge of what he looked like himself, as his diary notes. "To what extent is the loss of the image of the face connected with loss of the image of the self?" (25 June 1983).[2] Sometimes he would ask friends to describe a new person, especially if the person was a woman. Was she pretty? What was she wearing? This he would do even though he was aware of the many irrationalities inherent in this and asked himself why his feelings should depend on a visual appearance.

In those first three years he began to explore the voice far more and was amazed and excited to learn that for him, as for Peter White, all the emotion that is in the face is also in the voice. Intelligence, color, light and shade, melody, humor, grace, accuracy, laziness, carelessness, monotony, as well as vocabulary and precision of language, all became more important. Crucially though, he realized that he was far more passive, and depended on people disclosing themselves through speech. There were, for instance, no sneaky looks at a person when they were off guard. He continued to explore the consequences of loss of sight in minute detail. His diary entry of 17 September 1983 reads:

Nearly every time I smile, I am aware of it . . . aware of the muscular effort: not that my smiles have become more forced . . . but it has become a more or less conscious effort. It must be because there is no reinforcement . . . no returning smile . . . like sending off dead letters . . . I can feel myself stopping smiling . . . must ask someone if it is true.

He described the way in which his young family learned of the pointlessness of trying out their funny faces on Daddy and the way in which making love face to face no longer had the same significance. But above all was the centrality of the face as a defining icon of one's being. "The horror of being faceless, of forgetting one's own appearance, of having no face. The face is the mirror image of the self" (11 January 1984).

This is clearly an experience that neither Peter nor David could have been aware of. With this came a desire to hide his own face, desperate to find some equality, for if he could not see others' faces, why should they see his? He tried to hide his face with his hand. Around this time he found himself descending into a depression—writing of how blindness is associated in art with ignorance, confusion and unconsciousness. He would hide under a blanket, alone for hours on end, trying to find a place where solace was available.

Dreams became important—both dreams with sight and dreams where blindness was present, and even, bewilderingly, dreams where both states existed, dreams about anything, but most of all dreams with his family.

I had got out of bed . . . this toddler came padding in and I could see her quite clearly in the dim light . . . the first time I had been able to see her. I stared, full of wonder, taking in every detail of her face as she stood there, wreathed in smiles. "So this is her, this is the smile they all talk about." I had a wonderful sense of renewal of contact . . . then the dream faded. (21 August 1984)

As time went by he slowly left visual imagery behind. He described this as a very real journey.

The receding faces of Imogen and Marilyn [his daughter and wife] form a sort of fixed light at the far end, behind me. This provides a point of reference . . . to judge my traveling . . . It serves to exaggerate the time I have spent in the tunnel . . . as though during the first part of a journey through space the voyagers are aware of the speed with which they are parting from the still visible earth, but once out in the black vastness of space there is no longer the same sense of speed. As long as there is a receding image one is still aware of departing. Between that visual memory which mediates between us there is a deep black river of time, flooding the banks of my consciousness, carrying us apart. . .

I try to reconstruct my relationships on a new basis, yet i may be tempted to linger in the past, to indulge in the contemplation of your remembered image. (13 October 1984)

The only sighted world he had was historical, and this both offered comfort and threatened to dislocate him from the present, as it had Jeremy. He tried both to abolish the past and to find asylum in it. Intellectually he knew that he should forget his old sighted self and try to know himself on the basis of nonvisual data. The question was how this could be achieved, since he might not have any choice in the matter. Fortunately, not only did he know what the answer was but over the next few years he was able to come to terms with the reinvention of a whole new world which blindness imposed, and after four to five years reached a contentment and confidence. What he described as a long and lingering death, a period of intense personal mourning, was then over. In his own words he had gone from accident to meaning through an extraordinary journey of introspection.

In a very real sense the coming to terms with the loss of sight must be a journey that is beyond the imagination and, perhaps, comprehension of most sighted people. John Hull's book has provided enormous solace and inspiration to the blind. Its genius has been to give an insight into this passage to the sighted too. The book concerned the first few years after his complete loss of sight. What of the subsequent ten years now that he has had time to live in and assess his new world? I traveled up to Birmingham and, arriving early, wandered around the campus looking at the students. I went into the Barber Institute, a very fine art gallery. I lost a few hours in visual images before going into his department to see John.

I began by asking that if he had known he was going to go blind, would he have tried to store visual images?

"My loss of sight was very very gradual. The only time I could remember specifically doing that was when I was seventeen and my left eye no longer had sight and there was a curious moment when I realized I would no longer be able to see my left shoulder. I sort of said goodbye to it and knew that I would never be able to naturally see it again. As an adult I don't remember taking consciously one last look at my wife's face or at a photograph, probably because the deterioration in vision was so infinitely slow. I went through a period when I said to myself, I would never forget what so-and-so's face looked like, but I soon realized that was folly."

"What of the loss of the category of the face in terms of loss of the daily updating of the faces and expressions of those around you?"

"I can remember what my grandfather looked like, and my father and mother. I still find it easier to remember what the people look like whom I haven't seen since I lost my sight. In the case of those with whom my relationship with them has been continuous I have simply imposed my living relationship with them upon my old visual memory. My old facial memory is like that of an historian and I don't get it out."

This suggests that visual memory, memory now not replenished, is interfered with by updated verbally acquired memory.

"Of course I can remember what Marilyn's face looked like but only by recapturing particular moments, say when I met her off a train, when I can still sort of see her coming toward me smiling."

"Do you have a tactile perception, and appreciation, of the face?"

"It's a hard question. What does continually strike me is the lack of commensurability between what it looks like and what it feels like. You see my little boy's face, my five-year-old, is such a beautiful face, and often I touch it. He is a very robust boy, he would probably tell me to shut up if he heard me, but there is something curiously beautiful. I rest my hand lightly on his forehead at night sometimes, or I rest it over his face and the puckering of the childlike cheeks and nose and lips, and the fact that it's still small enough to be felt in the hand, somehow is curiously roselike. It is soft and flabby, there's a curious significance in all these nobs and little bits and pieces. It's a curious tactile thing that I don't think I ever enjoyed as a sighted person.

"This has developed. It wasn't described in the book. I've grown more sensitive to the blind state and to things about the face. Of course the thing about a blind person is that you cannot generalize because one's knowledge of faces is so concrete and intimate as a blind person. One doesn't sense the faces of many people and one doesn't want to. Occasionally, people ask me if I want to feel a face and on the whole I don't, but in women there is a curious oval quality about the female face, particularly their jaw seems to come to a point, whereas men's jaws are squarer, or so it seems to me. There is something so characteristic, effeminate in the feel of the oval of the female face, I don't know if that makes sense.[3] It excites me. There are a lot of erotic things about the face."

"How does one ever compensate for the lack of eye contact with the person that one loves?"

"That is still a perplexing thing for me but after years of adjustment I now do find that when feeling the curiously female bone structure or just running a finger along a bushy eyebrow, or feeling the soft part of the ear, I think I have been able to transfer a certain amount of erotic energy into tactile images of the face, which I never thought I would be able to do.

"For a long time I was deeply grieved over the lack of erotic excitement through the female face. I've never talked to anyone about this before because it has never occurred to me but I do believe that I have been quite successful in reestablishing it. Its range is very limited and it is significant that I have spoken about the face of a child and the face of a woman. What about the face of my male friends? I don't believe that I could—or would want to—have that knowledge of the face of male friends. There is something—tactility, or cultural, or just in me relating an intimacy to touch—something to do with tactility and pleasure. It took me a long time to transfer pleasure from the visual to the tactile. It is such a laborious ill-defined reconstruction, but I think that is what it is. The pleasure is from their face, not from their head."

"With your new friends, post blindness, how do you construct a personality without a face?"

"I no longer turn it into a visual image. I don't any longer know or care if they're tall, short, fat, thin, bearded, or what, don't give a damn. It doesn't occur to me to construct a physique through the voice. It takes time, more time perhaps. Everything is in the voice."

What was second, or rather *first,* nature for Peter White, John had to learn to do, constructing individuality from hearing.

"Do you say this person is like this because of his voice, say angry or sensitive?"

"Absolutely. I instantly know what my closest friends are thinking and feeling because its all in the voice—but they have to speak. There is a big problem with the child and the face. It's hard to tell moods. If my thirteen-year-old is taciturn a glance at his face would tell me how he was. Do you know what a dread I have? My fear is that my child would be killed or unconscious and I would be called to go to the hospital or the mortuary and identify my child *and I couldn't do it.* I would stretch out my hand and I would not know if it was my child or not. Or that I would be sitting beside my dead child, or my unconscious child, or my dying child, and I would not know, because it needs sight to know what the face under those conditions is doing. I might hold the hand but I wouldn't know what was happening because of an alienation from the face. When one of my children isn't feeling very well I stretch out my hand and say 'Well, you're hot, you're cold, you're clammy or sweaty.' I could tell those things, but all the subtlety, all the diagnosis of emotion of that child, experiencing whether the child is wan or pale, I can't tell, nor can I with Marilyn. I only have the voice."

"So, might your perception of emotional range have become different, narrower?"

"Anger, impatience, such emotions are more easily expressed in the voice than thoughtfulness or sadness. It is very difficult to detect sadness. The emotional range *is* narrowed. This is something I feel most acutely when I'm telling stories to my children and an even worse time is when I want to listen to music with them. That is an acute frustration. Telling stories is bad enough but listening to music is worse."

"I can tell a joke or share an experience several times with different sets of people and find it funny each time because they're renewing it through sharing."

"I'm not getting the feedback that allows that refreshment and rejuvenation. I would love my son Tom say to come and listen to a Beethoven violin concerto but he would be sitting there next to me and I have no way of knowing what it means to him. When it's finished I'd say at the end, 'Well what's it like?' and he'd say 'Great' and walk off and I still wouldn't know."

"Are you suggesting that the face expresses emotion in the finest way?"

"Exactly. And with music it's not what you say afterwards, it's the little glances that you show as it reaches its climax and you know you're in the music together and there's no fellow feeling without contact with the face.

"Now here's a big problem I've always had when I tell, say, a ghost story to my children. Its extremely difficult for me to know when I've gone too far because I don't see the quivering lip that tells you the next thing you're going to have is a scared child. And the same with humor. If you can see the face you can see that little wrinkling round the corner of the eyes that tells you that if you just push a little further you'll have a laughing smiling child. The blind person doesn't have that."

"You must live in a much more intellectual world."

"That's true absolutely. When I'm on a business committee all that matters is the business. The sighted people look around, someone's looking at some woman's legs on the other side, or there's a fly crawling up the coffee pot, or reading someone's notes under their papers or looking out the window, and there are you remorselessly chomping through it. I'm a marvelous chairman, once people get used to the technique. What I'm bad at is knowing when to back off. A sighted chairman knows when there is a sensitive area. I can sometimes pick it up when you get a feeling of tension in the room."

"One never normally consciously constructs character and feelings toward someone—it just happens. If you are more intellectual in approach these constructions may have required effort and thought and so have taken on a different aspect. I cannot imagine a character without a face."

"Marilyn and I have sweated blood on this one because it was so difficult for the sighted person to enter into that world. A year or two ago we had a visitor when Joshua was about three; when the friend had gone Marilyn said, apropos of nothing, 'What comes into your mind when I say Joshua?' I said, 'Well, Joshua.' And she said, 'What, what exactly is it?' 'Well, it's the memory running through my hand, the feeling, kicking, laughing body, of throwing him over my shoulder. Joshua's tummy when I put my hand on it in the bath and the things Joshua and I have done together.' 'Yes, but what of Joshua himself?' 'If you mean what does he look like—nothing.' 'I can't bear that, I can't bear to hear you say that because I feel that I'm closer to our friend who just left because she and I share the same Joshua.' I had to reply that I did not really know what she meant. 'Darling, but if we are going to say do we share the same Joshua, we might as well say "Do we share the same world?" and in saying "Do we share the same world?" there is a deep and important sense in which we do not. We do not share the same world.'

"Often I feel as if I am in another world but one can say this at a certain level and it's true but this is me being subjective. After all, the fact of the matter is that Joshua is a human being and Marilyn and I share the same person, love the same person, but in a different way."

"How do you view yourself?"

"A good question. I am not interested any longer in what I look like."

"But do you know what you look like?"

"I don't know what you mean by 'look like.' The category of 'looking like' has disappeared with me. I can remember passport photographs and things like that but they're irrelevant. Its like that with what Marilyn looks like. People sometimes say to Marilyn 'How lucky you are that John will not see you as you are getting older, never see the first gray hair.'"

"It annoys me to think that one can only appear beautiful at a certain age."

"That's right. And how awful to think that she would have an advantage through deceiving me. Sighted people assume that I will communicate with Marilyn through my nostalgic memories of the face and what she looked like ten years ago. When I explain to people that I do not want to communicate with the woman I love through a nostalgic detour, which now means nothing to me and is not related to my present relationship, they find that astonishing."

"But I see the photograph on the back of your book and she is beautiful, and then I think because she looks beautiful she must be beautiful and that's so deep within us. We, as sighted people, cannot escape the constant relationship between what we think people look like in facial terms and what the person is like underneath."

"Blindness is a great leveler. Occasionally I have a visitor from the Republic of South Africa and I can cause consternation by saying after a while 'Are you black or white?' Normally I know damn well from their accent but it disconcerts them that I neither know nor care."

Remembering David Blunkett's difficulties in thinking and disguising his thoughtful austere countenance, I asked, "Do you find that you have to think 'I must smile now because its expected?' Do you think a funny thought and think, 'Ah, now I'm smiling?'"

"That's such a good question. I am sometimes fearful that my face is becoming less expressive but Marilyn tells me this is not the case and that I have no need to worry about that but I feel it. I often feel that I'm thought to be too serious.

"It's hard for a blind person to have fun in a way because so much of the fun is visual, especially in the family. People making funny faces, teasing each other, and I can be out of it. It's so instantaneous, it can't be expressed in speech and I'm sometimes conscious of being heavy. I try to make up for that by hearing. Laughing together is one of the best things."

Normally, enjoyment smiles, social smiles, family smiles are all entwined, feeding off one another and creating new smiles. That was something John found difficult with and through the voice. "Do you smile on your own as perhaps you might have?"

"I am not sure. Not knowing about tears is worse than not knowing about smiling. Tears are silent. It's perhaps more important to know about tears than about smiles. Tears take longer, laughter is so ephemeral. I think there's no doubt that the loss of the face is a profound loss. A deeply dehumanizing loss. Having said that, the experience of living without faces does present another facet of human relationships which has its own adaptations and compensations."

"In speaking with you I am drawn to your face as I am to anybody else's."

"It's curious. It matters to me intensely whether people are looking at me when they speak or not. I can tell. I've got extraordinarily sensitive to that. It's the sound of the voice. I often say to my children 'Look at me' when I'm speaking to them."

"In fact I'm probably looking at you more intently because I want to pick up all the nuances."

"But don't you find it eerie that you are looking at the face of somebody who can't see you?"

"On the contrary. I may be taking advantage because I know I will not have to avert my gaze if you come back to me, but I don't find it eerie. I want to try and glean what I can from your facial expression and that's in a similar sense to anybody else who was sighted. I can maybe take more from you because I know you will not look back and we will not have to take turns in gazing."

"The lack of reciprocity doesn't bother you?"

"Well, I don't really feel that because you seem so alert and vibrant. Obviously having the eyes shut means that is a slightly dead area of the face. [The past eye operations have left John's eyes a little sunken and battle weary.] But your forehead is more expressive and you've got the big bushy beard."

"That's interesting. That has never occurred to me. You say my forehead is very expressive. I am anxious to be translucent because I am aware of the way in which blindness makes one invulnerable and I therefore have developed a style of total directness. My blindness exaggerates everything. It makes you more physical, makes you more spiritual, but you are on the stage in a spotlight. You can't see the audience but they are all gazing intently at you."

"Does that make you worried or feel vulnerable?"

"It used to bother me a lot, not having facial feedback from the audience bothered me an enormous amount. Now I don't give a damn. I've said what I believe and I say it as professionally and as well as I can—that's all I can offer. There is a certain distance in which one becomes indifferent to praise and blame because the distancing which blindness gives one removes one from that. I do care intensely but in a different way."

"You talk with so much exuberance and love and experience of your children. Does blindness make this more vivid, more precious?"

"Yes. Blindness makes one so minute, it makes one so particular. Not to have the face is partly a problem of the lack of imagination by the sighted person because the sighted person just cannot distinguish Joshua from the face. To say the word 'Joshua' and not evoke the face . . . "

"I am addicted to faces. Walking through the campus to meet you I had to look at everyone. People are inquisitive and particularly inquisitive about the face, and their perceptions of what a person is like are dependent on the face—we can't avoid that. We find a face on the moon, we find faces everywhere. Can you escape from that? Is it a release as well as a loss, a terrible loss?"

"In a way blindness is a purification of life. Whether that's true with other disabilities I don't know.[4] Possibly not so much, as much as blindness is—if you think of the way in which blindness has been treated in the mystical literatures. I am released in a way from the world of shopping, of television. Sometimes I feel I am looking at sighted people through a telescope and they look enormous, powerful, huge, wonderful, doing things I can't do—I can't imagine doing them—and that I'm missing out. Sighted people run the world, are busy doing things. Even at home sometimes Marilyn comes round and does something and I ask, How did you do that? 'Easy, I can see.' At other times I think I am looking at them through a telescope turned round the wrong way. They look like little ants busy with all the silly little things that won't make a scrap of difference to anyone, wasting their time away."

"But you once quoted Winnicott, 'To be seen is to exist.'"

"Yes, he talks about being in the presence of the face. He refers to the child seeing itself reflected in the mother. It occurs in scripture too. 'The Lord bless you and keep you: The Lord make His face to shine upon you . . .' Here I have a theological faith. There's another famous face in one of Paul's letters where he says that Moses had a veil over his face so that he could not behold the glory. One knows of the glory of God in the face of Jesus Christ, but there is no description of Christ. It is always said that no one could look on the face of God."

"Why?"

"Good question. You can hear the voice of God. One never knows what the face is like. It's never described, maybe because the face is such an indicator of the secretness of the individual, of the personality. It would be profane to have such knowledge of God."

"In the more austere forms of Islam, there is no representation of the face, not just God's face, anybody's face."

"Yes, that's true. Total rejection in the visual arts of representation, what does it tell us about the face in Islamic countries? I don't know. I think the word presence is very important because it's to be in *the presence of the face*. I nearly always find that when I'm in close contact with someone, deep conversation, that I need to touch them. Touch any part of them, not necessarily the face. Even with a man I would need to touch them. Maybe just on the hand (there is a sexual taboo as well), I wouldn't hold his hand, I would just lay my finger on it. Marilyn and I don't sit at opposite ends of the table; we sit together. Frequently I just put my hand down on the table and she'll touch it and it somehow makes up in part for not being in the presence of the face."

John's blindness has imposed on him an intensity—and yet through his family he retains an intimacy and humanity which he projects to others around him. It's almost as though the middle ground, the trivial, has been etched from his existence. Being with him taught me how to see—if not properly, then at least differently. I left John and went out into the sighted world again, having been unaware that for the previous few hours I'd been in a world of thought and of feeling and of intensity which had nothing to do with a visual world. Everything now seemed rather facile and thoughtless and immediate and trivial as I was distracted by light.

Both John Hull and Peter White were acutely aware of the possible isolating effect of blindness. Both, when talking with me, had returned again and again to their family. It was with their loved ones that they could sense moods and, by touch, know much that was lost to them in others. Blindness had imposed an intimacy. They were able to reach a full and rich emotional life through other channels of communication, but it was apparent that their blindness and particularly their loss of sight of the faces of others may have led to alterations in emotional range. It was talking with John that these losses following his blindness had become manifest, for his going blind had forced him to attend to matters which Peter had scarcely needed to consider consciously.

With John we had circled around two themes: the intellectual world and the feeling one, and the feeling world revolved around his children and wife in a very immediate, rich, and deep way. "What I love about my little boy is the way I just pick him up over my shoulder. The whole body is there. It is one of the things I love best. Although he's five he still has to be picked up at night. I just love going to his bunk bed at 10:30 or 11:00, yanking him out of bed onto my shoulder, holding his hand, loving the feel of him.

"There is something also about a woman's body which is extraordinarily expressive for a blind person, far more so than it ever was as a sighted person. A blind person doesn't know for most of the time what people are doing with their bodies. In the love relationship the curious thing is to have that knowledge of the entire positioning of the body, to feel somehow because of that one is in the presence of someone else, for so often as a blind person one does not feel in the presence of someone."

Peter White's experience was very similar. "One of the fascinations of children is that you can touch their faces. With my wife it's the feeling that you are entirely involved with someone at every level. The lights are not on and so there's no distraction for the other person. It's certainly important for me to have a family. I have two boys and a girl; the two boys were born first and my memories of them when they were small, and really that whole period from about two to three to about six or seven, when they are encompassable in a way, are enormously happy memories. There is a sort of completeness which, probably, all parents feel. Its a physical thing—they're small enough to be picked up. They could be played with and in a way you understand, or feel you understand, the whole of their life."

I had asked him if it was awful when they grow away in the sense they don't want to be touched.

"Yes, though oddly enough one did and one didn't. One of my sons, now twenty, an exuberant man, will come and jump on my back. Even with his mates around he'd come and kind of drape himself across me. My elder son is a bit more reserved but it was so much him that I didn't feel offended. With him I have a very talky sort of relationship."

As they grew up, I suggested, they changed physically.

"I am not concerned. That doesn't mean I am still picturing them as young. I'm not picturing them at all."

For Jeremy, three years after going blind, the category of "face," as the representation of self and of others, still has an importance, a centrality, even though for him it is so difficult to hold onto. John has been blind far longer and has traveled further, but despite this he still cannot forget.

"The person who cannot move the face has a curious kind of priestly witness—like a celebrant suggesting that all things are not necessary for human life. But you need to be an extraordinarily faceless person to accept that. Not to be in the presence of the face is a very profound loss."

Though the congenitally blind and those who have gone blind may appear to have a similar problem, it was soon apparent that there are huge differences in their approaches to the world in interpersonal communication and characterization. Peter White and David Blunkett, blind from birth, had not considered that they might be devoid of anything in either of these areas. The voice gave them most aspects and subtleties of mood and character—they used this to construct ideas of people which fascinated and engaged them as much as our visually dominated constructions. Though they may not be typical—both having chosen a "public" world—they do suggest, as Peter said, that if blind from birth, those parts of the brain concerned with sight get taken over to some extent by other senses, at least at a perceptual level.

In contrast, John Hull had an enormous—all but overwhelming—loss following the final, permanent, loss of his sight. His depression, and Jeremy's, were worst not when sight was lost, but when visual imagery began to fade. And it was that imagery of others and, in particular, that of the faces of loved ones, that was most difficult to accept. The loss of sight dislocated him from his family; no longer seeing their faces he no longer felt he could interact with them, be with them. Hull even questioned his own existence: "to be seen is to exist."

To be without sight leads us from the huge wash of faces met daily to a smaller but no less rich world. For the congenitally blind, character is constructed from voice seamlessly and unconsciously. For late-onset blind people this may be possible, but it may never be so easy to construct the character of others from voices or to think of oneself "residing in voice." If Hull's testament had shown the huge journey from the sighted social world to the unsighted one, and the centrality of the face and facial expression in that world, from Peter and David it was apparent that even for those who are congenitally blind there was something essential about the face. For them it seemed to represent a preferential part of the body, a site where attention in others was shown. At some level then, the face was buried within us, transcending sight and beyond experience. Having established this I went to those who could see but in whom there were various disconnections between what they took from the faces of other people and their sense of characterization. First, however, I needed to understand a little of the evolution of the face.

Bone to Brain

4

It is a most extraordinary thing that we have developed a small area of our bodies that is so expressive, so mobile, and so visible. I wanted to know how it had arisen and why. To look at the evolutionary pressures which led to its development meant looking at other animals and in particular at our nearest cousins, the monkeys and apes.

Thinking there might be clues from its use in nonhuman primates, I sought what was actually shown on the face of monkeys and apes. Animal ethologists, concerned with the study of behavior and action, talk of the face being a predictor and signaler of an animal's behavior. But might faces tell not simply of behavior but also of inner states? Perhaps if the origins of our own facial behavior could be understood from primates, then we might learn more about ourselves.[1] If our facial movements are innate predictors and displays of behavior then we might look at our selves differently than if our faces expressed inner states. On the other hand, such primate parallels might have been useful up to a point, but we might have left behind our evolutionary origin and replaced them with new and complex facial actions.

Fish Face

When the human fetus is five and a half weeks old and shaped like a bean, there appear from the underside three outgrowths. These branchial arches develop, in fish, into gills. In mammals, these buds of tissue merge and mix to form our forehead, face, and throat, with the second arch moving upward to form the face. The arches grow and move forward to fuse in the midline, forming an inner tube from which the gut and lungs develop.[2] In cold-blooded, "primitive," vertebrates the seventh cranial nerve innervates a large sheet of muscle covering much of the head, the constrictor superficialis muscle, lying over the lower aspect of the head and the neck. It acts relatively simply in respiratory function to open and close the mouth, eyes, and nose. Facial and head movement in such species, apart from breathing, is largely limited to biting, which has nevertheless become ritualized and used in threat.

In amphibians this single muscle layer is split into two, with the lower sheet breaking off to depress the jaw and the other layer wrapping round the lower face. In mammals the latter muscle splits in turn into a superficial platysma muscle and the deeper sphincter colli. Both of these migrate from the neck and throat toward the head and face during the evolution of the muzzle and then the face.

A further evolutionary step toward a face capable of expression and display may have required warm bloodedness.[3] This required insulation of the body from its environment; skin became softer and more malleable; hair, muscle, and nerve evolved to regulate the skin's posture and temperature. More mobile lips, cheeks, and hence faces were made possible by two further developments. Snakes tend to eat their prey whole; crocodiles kill it then tear bits off before swallowing them. In contrast, mammals chew their food more thoroughly before swallowing and, in primates, use the arms and forepaws to present it in manageable amounts to the mouth. Chewing requires more mobile jawbones, lips, and cheeks. Likewise, suckling in the young requires lips and cheeks. Mouths became more than entrances.

In parallel with these changes analysis of the world for these early mammals became dominated by a different sense. Early mammals, like the voles and field mice, find their way through the world largely by smell and by touch. They have long mobile hairs on their muzzles, moved by finely controlled muscles embedded at the side of the mouth and nose. In a few orders of mammals (the carnivores and the tree-living primates), the primacy of smell and touch sensation was superseded by vision, either to locate and attack prey or to enable movement in an athletically demanding habitat. To accommodate this the eyes became more forward facing (for improved binocular vision among other things). Once smell and touch were no longer the dominant senses, then large facial hairs were no longer necessary and the muscles controlling them were available for other movements of the face. These muscles became smaller, more delicate, and more finely controlled. Once vision dominated, the face was available to be seen by others. Thus a flatter, more forward-looking face, with few large hairs and a mobile lower face and lips, may have evolved, a face used to explore a visual world, and to eat, suckle, and vocalize. Parallel with these changes came the development of the front limbs. Once food could be manipulated and dissected by hands, a large jaw was no longer needed to catch and crush, and once the front limbs were manipulative, primates could rise from all fours onto their hind limbs. This allowed further development of the eyes, for the face was in a better lookout position. It was also presented more to the world—this face could be seen more by others. The more mobile it was, the greater its vocabulary. There is also some evidence that as the face evolved with a reduced jaw structure and mass, this may have allowed the development of a larger brain.

Communication between animals and species evolved to include vocalization and body posture. Later in evolution there were advantages in using facial display for this rather than the whole body. The face was more private, allowing communication to be directed at groups or even individuals, and it may have been more eloquent, allowing the development of a different, more refined, sort of body language. In fact, the development of the face as an unique identifier of members of the same species may have enabled development of a more refined sense of individuality itself than had been possible previously.

Darwin's Nose

The facial bones and skull are familiar to all from pirate flags, Hamlet, and innumerable photographs and drawings. In addition to their roles in jaw movement and respiration, the bones of the face also support the eyes and the organ of smell. But they also contribute to the face by setting the angle of the jaw, the height of the forehead, the closeness of eyes, and the contour of the face. A skull might be expected to suggest some aspects of a person, though in general a skull is not thought of as being individual in the way a whole face is. This receives a resonance—

though not any scientific support—from physiognomy, in which character is supposedly extracted from facial features dependent on the underlying skeletal structure, so that close set eyes are considered to go with untrustworthiness, and a strong jaw strength.[4] Darwin was almost turned down by Fitzroy, captain of the *Beagle,* because his nose was the wrong shape.

While there is no evidence of specificity of character as developed from facial features by the physiognomists, there is abundant evidence of the effects of medical correction of bony abnormalities of the face and skull. After such operations patients' lives may be changed.[5]

The Anatomy of a Smile

The origin of the muscles of the face from the branchial arches is reflected in their function and innervation. The temporalis and masseter muscles, two large muscles on the side of the head, are concerned with jaw stabilization and closing: they originate from the first arch and are innervated by the fifth cranial nerve, the trigeminal, which also supplies the face with sensation. All the other facial muscles are controlled by the facial, or seventh cranial, nerve, reflecting their common origin.

Early anatomists soon realized that dissection, which had enabled knowledge of the body's structure, did not allow for a good understanding of the muscles of the face. So finely embedded were they in the skin that removing the skin distorted and simplified the muscles underneath. The facial musculature could only be seen fully by studying the whole functioning face, which the neurologist Guillaume Benjamin Duchenne attempted with electrical stimulation in the nineteenth century. More recently, magnetic resonance imaging has allowed three-dimensional reconstruction of living moving anatomy. Gus McGrowther, professor of plastic surgery at University College, London, who has been active in this research, showed me some film of Billie Whitelaw, the actress, during a performance of Samuel Beckett's *Not I,* a play in which only the actress's mouth is lit. Her mouth and lips move continuously, in the most complex of ways, not just in smiling or pouting but in order to give the right intonation to the words. Yet these small sinuous movements modulating speech and respiration also visibly move the face and so allow facial expression.

In most muscles one knows function from anatomy. The biceps links the upper and lower arm bones—when it contracts, the arm bends; no one has won a Nobel prize for noticing that. Study of the richly innervated interweaving tissue of the face, however, might lead you to suspect a complicated use, but would not reveal its purpose. Most muscles in the body start and finish on bones, thus moving parts across joints. In contrast, while some muscles of the face often end at the bone, say at the angle of the eyes, many others begin and end within each other, forming a matrix of moving tissue independent of underlying bone and leading to complex relations between muscle shortening and facial movement.

With these provisos the muscles of the face may be divided into several groups: those concerned with the scalp, which allow elevation of the eye; those of the nose and mouth; and those whose action is intertwined with other muscles and so have less easily understood functions. The frontalis elevates the eyebrows when we look up, and in surprise. The muscle around the eye, the orbicularis oculi, which forms a circular band of decreasing radius, opens and closes the eye, both when blinking voluntarily and as a protective reflex. It also helps to release tears and raise or lower the eye at each corner. The superior portion contracts to wrinkle the midforehead just above the eye, in bright sunlight and when frowning. This description, however, taken from a textbook of anatomy, scarcely begins to convey all that this bundle of fibers does.

Within the orbicularis oculi the muscle's lateral and medial fibers are activated independently, as are those fibers close to and far from the eye itself. In a dust storm the outer fibers draw the eyelids shut like a purse string. In blinking the medial fibers contract more, bringing the lids inward toward the nose slightly. The eyelid can be brought either to or away from the nose, the cheek skin moved upward and laterally. Some of these coordinated movements, of the same muscle fibers in different combinations, are activated voluntarily; some are involuntary. "The eyes are the window of the soul." Everyone soon learns this. Yet a glass eye is as expressive as a real one—it is actually the muscles around the eye which give so much, or so little, away. How this is achieved and coordinated in various protective and expressive contexts is as yet poorly understood.

In comparison the movement of the nose might be considered simple. It has three main muscles: the procerus, which can wrinkle the nasal bridge during bright sunlight or frowning and mental concentration, and the nasalis and depressor septi, which dilate the nostrils. Even these are not solely respiratory muscles: Duchenne suggested they were the muscles of lust. Lower in the face are muscles which trace circular paths around the mouth: orbicularis oris and others, which go from the mouth to the lower jaw and cheek, to the ear, and to the eye. These act in concert to elevate and retract the upper and lower lips.

The modiolus, a small mass of muscle and fiber lying to the side of the mouth, complicates matters further. Nine muscles embed themselves in it. The modiolus prevents large movements of the lower face, which is the most mobile and least attached part of the facial musculature. It integrates activities of the mouth and cheek when biting, chewing, drinking, sucking, swallowing, speaking (including tone as well as articulation), shouting, crying, kissing, and, of course, the almost endless permutations of movements of facial expression. The risorius connects the outside of the mouth to the upper facial bone. When it contracts, the face lifts up and we smile, or we show pleasure, or appeasement, or love, or affection, or recognition, depending on context and individuality. The platysma and depressor muscles originating below the lips pull the mouth down and so help show sadness in a similar contextually driven manner. Some have attempted to explain facial expressions on the basis of the movement of individual muscles, while others have developed powerful techniques for analyzing movements of the face. Paul Ekman and Wallace Friesen in San Francisco have developed a facial action coding system that allows the description of facial movements in terms of the underlying muscle or muscles involved. It is astonishingly complex, with single-action units being active in many different expressions.[6] Such analysis allows some uncovering of what the face does, but even so the authors describe their work as "an approximation of the total repertoire."

The Vanity of Astronauts

The facial skin does not simply move according to the action of muscles inserted into it. It tells stories of its own, from the blushing young girl to the pimply adolescent boy (why is it the facial skin that is so affected during adolescence?). Its slow defeat by gravity reveals age far more than changes visible elsewhere on the body. Astronauts in space often take photographs of themselves early in their mission, because in zero gravity the wrinkles go. It is an expensive and temporary face-lift, since later in their mission fluid shifts can give them a slightly puffy look.

Facial skin may almost have evolved to tell others about our age and our past. The facial skin advertises health: a gray-blue discoloration around the eyes tells others how much sleep we have been enjoying. It has a memory and rarely lies, for it becomes wrinkled not only by age but by use. One blind woman, when asked how she found a man attractive, said that she felt around his eyes; if there were laughter lines then she knew more about him than from a short conversation. As Edwin M. Stanton said, a man of fifty is responsible for his face.

Bell's Nerve

The facial nerve supplies all the muscles of facial expression, branches going to each side of the face. As will be seen, complete paralysis of one side of the face follows damage to the facial nerve (Bell's palsy). Fortunately, most people recover from this damage, either because the nerve was not functioning but still intact, or because of regrowth. With regrowth, however, the nerve fibers do not always find their way back to the right muscle fibers. Occasionally, some nerve branches grow back to innervate muscles around the eye and the mouth. When this happens, the person may find himself or herself moving the mouth upward when blinking involuntarily, or winking when eating, an involuntary movement called synkinesis.[7]

For any accurate and controlled movement it is necessary to have feedback from the moving part. In the arms and legs there are nerve receptors, in muscles (muscle spindles), tendons and joints, which signal to the brain information about the position, movement, torque, and velocity of the part. Movement of the face is no less exquisitely accurate or controlled than that of the hands, yet no muscle spindles have been found in the facial muscles. Instead, feedback comes from the skin, which contains receptors very sensitive to stretch and movement, for it is not the length of a muscle fiber or the angle of a joint that is important in the face. Since skin movement and position are important for display, it is the skin that provides feedback.

Laughter and Sorrow

The facial nerve has direct connections to muscles of the face; when it fires they move. The facial nerve nucleus, in the brain stem at the top of the spinal cord, in turn is controlled from the brain and is directed to move by various parts of the brain under various circumstances.

Complete paralysis of one side of the face can occur with facial nerve damage and following a stroke in the cerebral cortex on the opposite side of the brain. Paucity of facial movement is seen in people suffering from Parkinson's disease, affecting an area of the brain called the basal ganglia. In those with Parkinson's there may be reduced facial expressiveness on both sides of the face, though if you startle them or ask them to move their face voluntarily, movement is relatively preserved. It is the involuntary, instantaneous facial movements that are reduced. In contrast some persons with cortical brain damage, a rare occurrence, are not able to move their faces voluntarily, but can effortlessly move them according to mood—the reverse of the situation in Parkinson's.

While some patterns of facial movement appear to be under both voluntary and involuntary control others are seen only with genuine feeling states. The activation of the orbicularis oculi around the outside of the eye tends to occur with enjoyment smiles but not with social smiles.[8,9] This may reveal the origins of these expressions: in monkeys "appeasement" smiles and "enjoyment" smiles are more clearly differentiated. This in turn agrees with what is common knowledge, namely, that we can "make" faces in social situations but usually never completely disguise our feelings, though poker players and politicians might disagree.

Both cerebral motor cortex and basal ganglia may be fairly low in the level of command of movement of the face. So called higher centers may control when and how much we make faces. Evidence for this comes from careful experiments involving stimulation of the brain, in conscious people, prior to surgery for epilepsy (this maps which bit of the brain controls which movement, and allows the surgeon to avoid operating on the more important areas if at all possible). Arroyo and colleague studied people with fits of a very unusual sort: laughing, or gelastic, epilepsys.[10] When they stimulated the brain of one subject she laughed but without any internal feeling of mirth. Two other subjects had fits accompanied by both laughter and mirth. The authors concluded that an area of the brain called the frontal anterior cingulate area might be involved in the motor act of laughing, but the basal temporal area was involved in its emotional appreciation. So there may be some dissociation in the brain of areas involved in the generation of acts of laughter and sorrow on their face, and their perception by the individual.

Cars and Faces

Any consideration of perception of faces must involve discussion of how other people's faces and facial displays are recognized, as well as feedback of one's own face. Faces are, after all, designed to be seen: a face is often the first thing we see as babies and our memory for faces is huge.[11]

Early analysis of vision occurs in the posterior part of the cerebral cortex, in a part called the occipital lobe. A lesion in the occipital lobe causes complete blindness. But it is the more selective and subtle deficits in visual perception that we are concerned with here—rare syndromes in which vision is intact except for deficits in the recognition of faces as described in *The Man Who Mistook His Wife For a Hat*.[12] It seems incredible that we might lose perception of familiar faces, a disorder called prosopagnosia. Does this tell us about how important faces are for us (that there are areas of the brain solely devoted to faces), or do such people also have subtle problems in other aspects of visual recognition?

Despite their notoriety, subjects with prosopagnosia are rare, occurring a few at a time in the medical literature. Sergent and Signoret studied four such persons, and compared their perceptual deficits with scans of their brains.[13] One of their subjects was defective in all aspects of face processing, being unable even to realize that two identical photographs of the same face were the same individual. Yet he could identify car makes, models, and years as a normal person would. Another subject could not recognize faces as belonging to someone, but was still able to understand the expression or emotion any given face was displaying. The damage to the brains of the patients was quite large, making accurate localization of function difficult. But patients with the most severe and least selective face-processing deficits had damage to the right side of the brain, in the occipital cortex and the posterior part of the medial temporal lobe. The subject who could recognize emotion but not physiognomy had damage further forward in the brain, in the anterior temporal cortex and parahippocampal areas.

The arcane details of cortical processing of the face need not concern us, but the general principles and layout are of importance. Facial information is processed mainly in the right hemisphere. The "simpler" types of prosopagnosia may reflect damage posteriorly in the brain, near the primary visual cortex; more complex deficits in perception of faces and emotion may be associated with medial temporal and frontal damage. The frontal lobe may be involved in expressiveness and the temporal area, together with the subcortical limbic and hippocampal areas, in the experience of emotion.

Science often progresses by separating variables in order to analyze them. Of course the movement acts of expressing sorrow and its experiencing usually coexist inseparably. But one deficit may affect another function. Some people with Parkinson's have difficulty in both expressing "emotional" faces and in recognizing them in others and, more surprisingly, in *imagining* emotional faces.[14] Thus loss of or reduction in facial movement in a person may lead not only to difficulties in recognizing facial expression in others but also to problems in imagining such emotional faces, showing interactions between motor acts and their feedback at many levels. If nothing else, the neurological work has shown just how much of the brain is involved in the movement of facial muscles and in the perception of that movement.[15] After that the question of what the face does would seem simple, but as we will see, that was before people started thinking about it.

Chimpanzees' Dreams

5

If we have an understanding of how the face evolved in animals, then the next thing to consider is what exactly facial display communicates in nonhuman primates and in humans, for it is clear that faces in these groups—and in particular in ourselves—do new things, things not apparent in other species. The evolutionary pressures that led to our face might tell us something of the factors that led to the emergence of humans. To what extent might we, as a species, be understood by our faces?

I sought to answer these questions by looking at the use of faces and facial expressions in nonhuman primates. There was agreement about much of this, but the scientific writing seemed devoid of a sense of monkeys and apes as individuals, which the face in part seemed to allow. So as well as reading I went to talk with zookeepers about their primates, for they should know their charges as well as anyone. That led me, by a circuitous route, to psychoanalysis. First though, I wanted to know what others had thought that faces actually did.

From Aristotle to Darwin

What facial language communicates has been the object of consideration since the time of the Greeks. Aristotle believed that facial displays in humans are characteristic patterns related to clearly identifiable internal emotional states recognized by others.

Everyone knows that grief involves a gloomy and joy a cheerful countenance . . . There are characteristic facial expressions which are observed to accompany anger, fear, erotic excitement and all the other passions.[1]

Aristotle made the implicit suggestion that facial displays carry a valence or feeling in themselves when he wrote of "a gloomy" countenance. Part of what gloom means is a facial movement. Aristotle was enunciating what might be termed a commonsense rule: faces express "passions" or emotions. Man has surely developed such a mobile and expressive face, far beyond that seen in the apes, because of the refinement of emotions. Charles Bell,[2] in the early nineteenth century, took this a little further, thinking that the violent passions were marked on the face of both humans and animals by movements of muscles specifically designed by the divine for that purpose. He distinguished states of mind—introspective thoughts—from emotions or passions, and almost defined the latter in facial terms.

Duchenne,[3] a few years later, studied the face using two comparatively new and exciting techniques: electrical stimulation of the facial muscles and photographic recording of the resultant "expression." He became fascinated by his experiments and produced a series of astonishing photographs, one of which is in the Museum of Modern Art in New York City. He concluded that some muscles could produce fully formed facial expressions on their own, whereas others produced expression only by working with others in various combinations or blends. He ranked muscles in order according to their importance in producing expressions. The forehead muscles were the most important, muscles which today are considered the most difficult to "fake." He gave muscles titles according to their function. This he wrote of the muscle of attention (frontalis in the forehead), and the muscle of lust (the part of the nasalis at the side of the nose). Though we may not agree with all his conclusions, his work is a most amazing journey into the face and the mind. For Duchenne,

Once this language of facial expression was created [by God], it sufficed for Him to give all human beings the instinctive faculty of always expressing their sentiments by contracting the same muscles. This rendered the language universal and immutable. . . . To express and monitor the signs of facial expression seem to me to be inseparable abilities that man must possess at birth.[3]

Duchenne, like Bell, observed the Creator's work and marveled at His expertise. On the other hand, Charles Darwin—not a renowned churchman—turned his attention to the face while writing *The Descent of Man,* which placed man close to our fellow animals. Whereas Bell had been descriptive and deductive, and Duchenne experimental, Darwin, through these techniques and more, had a thesis to prove: that facial displays were genetically inherited. It would then follow that the most human of characteristics, the face, might be brought into an evolutionary framework like the rest of our being. Darwin scoured the literature—and the world—for evidence. Though acknowledging the previous masters, Duchenne, Bell, Lavater, and many more, he also acknowledged the many people who replied to his letters pleading for information on people not exposed to Western culture.[4] He considered evidence from the expressions of animals, from children, from the congenitally blind, from the insane, and from art. He visited zoos, putting a living freshwater turtle in with monkeys to see if they expressed surprise (their eyes opened widely, their eyebrows moved up and down, and their faces lengthened).

Darwin wanted also to understand the semiotics of facial expression—why certain movements communicate certain emotions. For unlike much spoken language, in which the word may not have a relation to the fact (except for onomatopoeic words), he felt that with the face there must be some such link. He did find commonality of facial display, not only between man and primates but in all mammals, suggesting that they had arisen from more primitive uses of the face. He thought that our facial displays came from preadaptive movements which had been used by our ancestors during respiration, and which had come to represent emotions, as those emotions themselves, and their expression, had evolved from more primitive functions.

During weeping, for instance, he wrote, the eye is closed and tears flow, a response that originally protected the eye from the raised pressure and engorgement of the blood vessels associated with screaming. Frowning was the result of being able to control a crying fit, with some contraction of the brows remaining. Other expressions defeated him. He did not know why with low spirits the whole face falls and the features become lengthened. He could not suggest why such a complex movement existed for the sole purpose of expressing grief. He also realized that other emotional states, "jealousy, envy, avarice, revenge, suspicion, deceit, slyness, guilt, vanity, conceit, ambition, pride, and humility" were not revealed by facial expression. He may have taken solace in quoting Shakespeare who, in writing of envy as "lean-eyed" or "black" or "pale," accepted that he too was unable to find correspondence between feeling and the face for some emotions. Just as he could not explain all the semiotics of expression—the relation of facial movement to meaning—so he still had trouble in understanding how some expressions developed. Bell and Duchenne had invoked the Almighty. Darwin's explanation was scarcely less fantastic given his development of evolution by natural selection:

Every true or inherited movement of expression seems to have had some natural and independent origin. But when once acquired such movements may be voluntarily and consciously employed as a means of communication. The tendency to such movements will be strengthened or increased by their being thus voluntarily and repeatedly performed: and the effects may be inherited. (p. 355)[4]

The use of Lamarckian principles to explain the inheritance of facial displays and their relation to expression of emotion came after his great book on evolution was published. Why did he have to resort, uniquely, to Lamarck to explain this? Montgomery has suggested that Darwin was guided by the teaching of his grandfather Erasmus, who subscribed to the theory of association, whereby actions of different muscles—once connected by habit—then tend to move together subsequently.[5] Yet this, and the desire to disprove Bell, do not seem quite adequate. Perhaps, as Montgomery suggests, Darwin tended to use natural selection for morphological change and the inheritance of acquired characteristics for behavior in which case he may have underestimated socially learned factors and did not realize how those parallel mechanisms for change, natural selection, and culture, might be brought together.[6]

Universal Faces

More recently Paul Ekman, C. E. Izard, and others, have provided further evidence in support of Darwin.[7] Their techniques have been comparatively simple in concept though very complicated in execution. They have shown photographs of facial expressions to peoples in different cultures and determined whether a facial expression signifies the same emotion to people all over the world. Their photographs of the expression of certain emotions (anger, happiness, fear, disgust, sadness, and surprise) were shown to people in America, Brazil, Japan, Argentina, and Chile, who were asked to choose the most appropriate single-word description of the emotion from a list of six (anger, happiness, fear, disgust, sadness and surprise once more). They found very high levels of correspondence between cultures for the six emotions: above ninety-five percent for happiness, down to around sixty-five percent for a picture of fear. All these cultures had been exposed to modern media, so next they went to Borneo and New Guinea to conduct similar experiments on a group of preliterate peoples who could not have been contaminated by Western culture.[8] Once more the choices of emotion were high: above ninety percent for happiness and down to sixty-eight percent for surprise. From such experiments the authors developed the neurocultural theory of facial expression. Some expressions were considered learned and culturally determined, but some emotions and the expression of these emotions were universal and thus likely to be innate, as Darwin had thought.

If some emotions were expressed on the face and some not, then the facial ones might, in some way, be special. Some people have subsequently defined emotions partly in terms of facial display (a pleasingly circular argument), and even suggested that these facial expressions reveal something basic about human nature itself.[9]

Culture and Colors

Two human characteristics not revealed simply on the face are doubt and iconoclasm. Recently, several groups have questioned much of the evidence on universality and cast doubt on the concept itself. Others have questioned if the states of mind shown on the face are discrete emotions, and wondered whether some emotions can really be more basic than others. The academic arguments have relevance because in dissecting what we do with our faces all seem to agree that they are approaching what we are about and whence we came.

Anger, aversion, courage, dejection, desire, despair, hope, hate, love, sadness, disgust, wonder, guilt, grief, expectancy, and shame—Ortony and Taylor noted that few authors could agree on which emotions were basic.[10] Some, like surprise, Ortony and Taylor doubted could be termed emotions at all. An emotion, they suggested, required—and was defined by—an affective valence, that is, the person had to experience a positive or negative feeling. Surprise was valence neutral, until the surprise was overtaken either by happiness at a pleasant surprise, or fear or sadness at an unpleasant one. Fear, in fact, is the expression most often confused with surprise, presumably because surprise (at the unknown) most often merged with fear in our ancestral environment. Interest, similarly, was a cognitive or thinking state, rather than an emotional or feeling one leading you to find out more.

The face is not up to signaling all this. Maybe, instead, there are biologically based, inherited, basic "emotions," or "drives." Panksepp has written of three such systems, one for exploration or expectation and desire; one for flight, fear, and horror; and a third for offense, anger, and rage through sadness, crying, and sorrow, to grief and panic.[11] Some of these might be seen in animals, but some seem inherently rather more human or primate. Gray in turn has talked of systems for fight and flight (rage and terror), positive emotions, (joy, even perhaps, love), and a behavioral inhibition system, associated with anxiety.[12] These are biological, basic, in the sense that we can see some animals behaving according to drives similar to those which may motivate us, a long way from the "basic emotions" associated with the face.

Ortony and Taylor discussed anger, a prototypic emotion, in terms not of a basic expression, but as a blend of several other displays. The furrowed brow might accompany frustration or puzzlement; the open set mouth, preadapted attack; the compressed lips, resolve; the raised upper eyelids, increased vigilance and attention. Each expression, even the so-called basic ones, might in fact might be made up of subcomponents. This led Putchnik to suggest that basic emotions combine like a child's paints on a palette.[13] Sometimes a red and yellow will each remain recognizable in orange, but sometimes yellow and blue will be chosen to yield a completely unexpected color.

As can well be imagined, Ekman and Izard have made robust replies to these articles.[14] In some cases the data allow for differing interpretations. Attempts have been made to compromise, since after all Ekman has always called his theory neurocultural, agreeing that many facial displays are cultural, while the behaviorist-cultural workers do not dispute that some facial expressions are recognized at above chance levels by most people, and so may be genetic. One has the feeling that the groups are debating more than data interpretation and experimental design. Both seem to understand how differently we may be forced to view ourselves if we see culturally learned rules on the face rather than universal, ancient and innate evolved meaning. At least both groups talk of emotions and facial expressions in the same breath.

Smiling Happy People?

In contrast, some groups have dismissed ideas of facial *expression* at all and talk instead of facial *display*. Fridlund provided evidence for facial actions being part reflex, from schematization of signals seen in more primitive animals, and part social.[15] He describes the facial displays of reptiles (an open mouth, with or without teeth baring), and the facial displays of greeting, grooming, submission, and threat seen in fur seals and walruses. He suggests that some facial behaviors become formalized into displays from two types of movement: intention movements and facial reflexes. The former often precede action, for example, lip retraction before attack. The facial display then becomes a substitute for the action having derived directly from the truncated movement.[16]

Facial reflexes in turn are usually protective, for instance, blink following irritation of the eye. Disgust may arise from the gag reflex seen with something touching the back of the throat.[17] Complex displays may involve both primitive reflexes and instrumental habits. For instance, the facial display for threat involves direct gaze (which may be protective), and a tightened jaw, which may be an intention movement associated with attack and biting. If facial displays are not readouts of feeling states or emotions, but rather are tools for organizing social interaction, then it follows that they need not be used all the time, but only when a social interactant can be influenced. Children smile not when they open a present but when they turn to their parents; adults' joy at a strike at tenpin bowling is shown not when they are pointing downlane at the pins, but when they turn to their friends. Lovers smile during courtship but not during coitus. Fridlund writes:

Although adults can surely experience emotion, the relation of adult display to emotion is adventitious. Displays serve social motives, which themselves depend little upon emotional state. We may be courteous, loving, amusing, or reassuring, and smile accordingly, if we are so moved—regardless of whether we feel happy, sad, angry or fearful. I know of no evidence that we smile more when we are happy. . . .[15]

Thus we should use few facial displays while on our own. This is the case, but we do still make some, and this fact has been used by those who think that facial displays are readouts of emotion. Fridlund rejects this by suggesting that even when alone we imagine others are present, or rehearse for when we will meet people, or even treat inanimate objects or pets as interactants. It seems unlikely, however, that when we are alone all facial expressions can be so explained. Stronger emotions at least seem to be expressed regardless of interactants. Consider when we are walking alone and see or smell something bad; our faces will register disgust. If we are rock climbing alone and slip, we register fear. Fridlund's thesis, that emotional expression is a social display, may be correct in that we exaggerate weaker expressions for social purposes, but the stronger ones seem secure regardless of context and audience.[18]

Though reducing facial movement to social display, Fridlund still acknowledges that most people see them as facial expressions of inner emotions. Perhaps this has arisen from etiquette; "I feel angry," is more acceptable than "I'm going to attack you." Suggesting feelings is refined, stating intentions is brazen. We rarely find out if another's face and social motives are matched by the expected emotion; we seldom, for instance, ask smilers if they are happy or not. Fridlund thinks the continued existence of an emotional view of facial expression is due to a Rousseauan romanticism, a belief that emotional faces signify authenticity and personal integrity, whereas social faces reflect an inevitable loss of innocence forced by society. Darwin had set out to place facial display in an evolutionary context, to put us, even in one of our most human of characteristics, at the head of the line of the rest of the animal kingdom. The work of Fridlund and other neo-Darwinians appear to have buried us, and our faces, more and more in a world of facial display and social manipulation. Is there a way out of this, back to an Aristotelian world of emotion and facial expression? Surely we are doing more than divining motive and predicting action when we look at faces? In an attempt to answer these questions I went to talk with primatologists, for if they saw more on the face of their animals than readouts of behavior, perhaps our facial expressions had evolved beyond manipulation and display too.[19]

Decoding Primate Faces

If a certain face is always followed by a certain behavior, it seems reasonable to suggest that the facial display is intentional. Alternatively, if an animal's face does not always look the same in similar situations and if the previous behavior or physical condition of the animal is important, it suggests the face may be expressing more complex inner states. We need initially to know how facial display corresponds to behavior.

Van Hooff described a number of facial displays in monkeys and apes which could be separated and decoded, some with rigid behavioral contexts, some not. [20] The tense-mouth face, with widely opened staring eyes and eyebrows lowered in a frown, mouth and lips closed, precedes and accompanies an attack. A second face, with the eyes staring, eyelids apart, eyebrows lifted, ears retracted with the teeth bared, is seen both with attack and the threat of attack, and with flight or grooming. Characteristic vocalizations (low-pitched grunts or barks) and body posture (jumping movements) accompany it, all three channels being used together. In response to attack the staring bared-teeth scream face may be seen (a display Darwin described as terror). The whole face is mobile, with ears back, eyes fixed on the opponent, eyelids apart, eyebrows lifted up, mouth open, and teeth bared. High-pitched staccato barks are emitted. It usually precedes fleeing, but there can be conflict between that and a returned attack, and when the animal is frustrated.

These faces may seem fairly stereotyped and clearly related to action. Others are less related to external events. Van Hooff draws attention to the neutral face, seen in all monkeys when lying around or sitting. Though not accompanied by action it shows relaxation and disengagement. The alert face, with eyes fully opened and with increased tone of the facial skin, is shown during grooming, mounting, and even some flight. It does not signal an action but is displayed in a context defined by situation and by a relationship between two individuals. In the silent bared-teeth face the eyes are directed at the opponent either in a fixed way or in short glances. The performer might avoid, or flee, or approach and then embrace or play. Rarely the observer might attack, though more usually he or she adopts behavior similar to that of the performer, and a relationship based on facial display is entered, faces being used to alter behavioral states in one individual by another according to context.

So, while some facial displays are unambiguous and predict behavior, others depend on context, including mutual gaze itself.[21] Some are invitations to share; others are associated with shifts in levels of alertness. They may be displays and *conversations* between individuals. This suggests the need by observers to take into account other individuals, so that these displays might depend on the animals' past relationship and inner levels of alertness at the time, things beyond the animals' actions. But the primate literature is concentrated on those facial displays which are clearly related to behavior; I wanted to investigate the grayer areas of idiosyncrasy and interpersonal relationship, thinking that held the key to the emergence of such an expressive face in humans. I had to find people who knew a few nonhuman primates well. It was time for the zoo.

Howlett's Zoo, Kent

Howlett's Zoo in Kent has a collection of small primates and a society of gorillas. I wandered around with the keepers one very hot July day. As we went up to small groups of lemurs, langurs, and gibbons, they came to greet us, coming to eye or chest level to have a look. Some of their faces were almost immovable despite their inquisitiveness, while other species had the most rapid indecipherable flashings across their faces, eyelids, foreheads, mouths, and cheeks moving rapidly in ways I could neither keep up with or begin to analyze.

Ernie Threlfall, their keeper, had little idea of what to make of their facial displays either, though he had been around nonhuman primates for years. He had been taught not to look at them while in the cages, to avoid threat, and most days he was too busy to stand and watch from the outside. He did, however, remember some occasions when he was privy to facial behavior. A banded langur was trying to wean an infant after three and a half years. The baby was kicking and spluttering. One day when Ernie was in the cage the mother came up to him and, quite unprompted, looked at his face and then at the baby. He is sure she was saying "help me." Another monkey had evidently had a hard time and was psychologically unbalanced, as many are in captivity. Her face was tense and showed suffering. Ernie was amazed that when she was very ill her face relaxed so much that she was almost unrecognizable. A chimpanzee he looked after used to be aggressive and anxious both in her body and facial posturings. He couldn't work out the trigger until he realized it was her estrus cycle; she had premenstrual tension.

Ernie introduced me to a pair of gray-faced gibbons. The female came up to us at chest level, looked at us, and then, looking away, offered Ernie her arm through the cage, like a shy Victorian lady. He took it and then she did the same to me. I moved, but Ernie stopped me, explaining that he could not predict her behavior. They had just put the pair together to mate but the male had beaten her. She was seeking our reassurance, while the male was at the other end of the cage. It turned out that he had been attacked by other males previously and had taken it out on her. I looked across at the male, sitting on a branch, and saw his lips tense. Was that a known facial display in gibbons, I asked Ernie? Not as far as he was aware. I wondered whether it was a display at all, in the sense of needing an knowledgeable observer, or a spillover of an inner emotional state.

It was so hot the gorillas were sleepy. I talked with Peter Halliday their head keeper, and with a Japanese ethologist, Naoby Olcayasu. In gorillas the great forehead ridge is the most expressive part of the face, together with eye gaze. They look at others out of the corner of their eye, to avoid direct stare and hence threat. Sometimes they might be making a face and displaying something unwanted, so they look away to conceal it.[22] As we talked the great silverback, the boss, was keeping an eye on them all, while the others were looking around with the corners of their eyes. The silverback's huge brows were moving slowly in the sunshine. Down at the corners, Peter explained, meant submission. They all yielded it to the silverback. He, in turn, yielded once a week on a Sunday afternoon, when John Aspinall, the owner of the zoo, fed them from a walkway above the cage.

Monkey World, Dorset

It was evident from Howlett's how different nonhuman primate species were in their use of facial expression. But I could not grasp the relation between facial mobility, intelligence, and individuality. Maybe the langurs were bright; they certainly looked it. But then so were gorillas with less facial movement. Maybe another variable was the complexity and stability of their societies and the opportunity to show their faces to others. One, the closest species to us, and with the most mobile of faces, is the chimpanzee.

Monkey World, a primate refuge in Dorset, was set up in 1987 for primates rescued from circuses and beach photographers. These animals, captured in the wild and often seeing their mothers and elders killed in the process, cannot be released into the wild again. Having been traumatized or taught to smoke or clap to command, often having been drugged and half-starved, they would not last long. Jim Cronin took over Monkey World in 1991. He had taken a few degrees, worked in the Bronx Zoo—and been fast-tracked as a curator there—when he upped to "join the circus." He ended up in Britain, at Howlett's, transfixed to see the way Aspinall got into the cages with his gorillas, respecting them, loving them. He stayed for seven years before moving to Dorset. Since then he has been running Monkey World as an asylum for chimpanzees, orangutans, and some smaller primates.

I walked around the site with him and his curator, Jeremy Needall. There are three large enclosures for chimpanzees, each with about nine individuals in four acres or so. Jim and Jeremy explained that the groups were quite stable despite the unusual way they had been formed. A dominant alpha male emerged in each group, though if young and unsure he would bully. Older, more mature alpha silverbacks maintained order by personality.

We saw one group at play in the sun. I asked about the face, voice, and body language. They were agreed it was all three together, but that it was often very quick and subtle. Jim pointed out Sammy, "Sammy will throw rocks at you, even with a relaxed face. I don't think he's evil or deceiving. That is just him. He does what he enjoys." Like Buster Keaton, I thought (though Keaton's poker face may have originated when he was used as a "human ball" in vaudeville as a child and made not to show the pain he was enduring). We sat down next to the wire of a large enclosure (Jim doesn't often go in with the monkeys, wanting to give them their own space). I said that when watching the chimps they had never looked back into my face. Jim replied, "You have to remember that they see lots of people. They are not stressed. Unless you do something for them, why be attentive?"

They came up to Jim, who had crouched down and was alternately looking down and looking at the chimps he knew. They came up to him hooing and greeting. They were interested in Jim because they knew him. Occasionally one would get excited, and so would the rest for no obvious reason. "There's Charlie. He's not taking part. I don't know what his mental state is or where he is most of the time." Charlie was an older chimp and looked it. He looked sad in his whole posture, in his face, and in his apparent isolation from the group. A small bright eyed chimp came up to us. "This is Athena, the baby of the group. She can get away with anything for they all look after her. She's an ex-circus chimp so she will walk round doing the tongue-out smiling-chimp stuff, clapping hands."

Jim and Athena were by now marching up and down each side of the wire, imitating each other, looking at each other, each yelping in delight. Athena was pulling faces the whole time, faces the others did not seem to be doing. Jim went on, "They sneak, say in sexual behavior. One male last year goes up a tree with a female chimp he shouldn't. So he's looking around trying to be nonchalant about it, very humanlike. The interesting bit was not so much that, but the chimp that ratted on him. This chimp did not say much but he looked across at the silverback and then looked up. Paddy (the silverback) looked back at him and then looked up. As Paddy looked up, the chimp went as though to say, 'Look at that!' and ratted on him. Paddy went up the tree after the first chimp and there was trouble, big trouble. But the chimp that ratted was saying, 'I can't have her, so neither can you.' It had to be intent because he guided his eyes. Then he joined in and chased and beat up the errant male."

Both Jim and Jeremy played with their animals and had built up relationships, having got to know each chimp. Jim explained that the best people to sit and know what the chimps would do were children. They could get inside. Eight- to nine-year-old children had the imagination and were working out relationships and a whole host of social rules which we as adults had been dulled to, and were able to predict actions in another species more easily because of it.

I walked to another enclosure with Jeremy. If Jim is fast, enthusiastic, and garrulous, Jeremy is more measured and solid (a chimp to an orang). "Life is simple; their body language is simple, though there are many dialects. I need a relationship between me and the chimps. In some it is love-hate; in others love-love. Take Paddy the dominant male; it took me three years to get any physical contact with him, and now if he is in the right mood we will sit and chew the fat, in a quiet private manner if nobody's looking, 'cos he's dominant male and so am I. Sometimes he will want a tickle, sometimes not."

I explained my feeling that facial display in nonhuman primates involved not only predictors of behavior—like the fear-grin face—but also other expressions which were more individual and depended on mood.

He agreed. "This is the reason I do what I do. The more experience I get, the more I realize that it would be so much easier to quantify if I had only been doing it for a couple of months. Now I am afraid of making it *too* individual. I have to speak 39 different languages. We put on so many fronts, much of our social interaction is defensive or trying to coerce, because we meet so many people. But in chimps they may meet only forty or so. There are lines drawn, particularly in submissive gestures. The risk is that if I do turn my back, I will misjudge mood and end up with fang marks."

I suggested that we all take risks when we reveal our feelings.

"If I know an individual well, then I can decide whether to leave the individual alone, or go to tickle him. I may have got it wrong, but that is the risk I take. There is no way if you introduced me to a group of your chimps that I, as a stranger, would be anything but submissive. I would look at my feet and so forth. Chimp/human relationships usually take a lot longer than human ones."

These relationships were based on mutual knowledge and reading, not only of behavior but also of mood. It was clear that this was what Jeremy and his charges were doing, in their own idiosyncratic way.

We had walked over to a pair of orangs.[23] They are supposed to be asocial creatures, who live in near isolation but who can recognize individuals very well. They have nearly impassive faces, for why move a face if you live alone? As we walked up to them, the male, Benji, somersaulted onto a net and gave Jim a big smile. He anticipated my question. "To see if I was interested. Orangs are difficult to figure out, because they do not do a lot with their face; in fact he may not tell you much when he's chewing your arm off. A chimp does more; a lion does nothing. You can watch orangs for a long time and see nothing, and then see at least four facial expressions all at once. They will work on particular problem for months. If a chimp can't do it immediately, they give up. Say a long twig to reach something, or a small weakness in the wire. Orangs are great problem solvers." One day Benji had taken a stick, dipped one end in water and while holding the other end, which was still dry, had given it to Jim through the electrified perimeter wire. Unwittingly Jim had taken it and got a shock. Benji smiled, but wouldn't take the wet end. Jim laughed too—afterward. "They are more solitary and more interesting. You don't get a fast instant reaction. I can wind all these chimps up very fast simply by moving or joking. But if I do that with the orangs they will look at me and think I am a jerk. We can't turn them on or off so easily, so ethologists often go off and study something else."

It was apparent just how easily chimpanzees were turned on and off. They constantly had to be aware of their position with other chimps. I had seen them in stable enclosed communities; in the wild, groups altered, making it more complex, more bewildering for individuals to keep their position and predict others' behavior toward them, like new kids in a playground. Gorillas and orangs established more stable groups and were subsequently less at risk, so was it coincidence that their facial displays and whole behavior were more measured? By now Jim was asking Jeremy what any chimp might gain from being more facially expressive. "That depends on character. Nobody messes with Paddy. He is about the most antisocial chimp I have met, but he wants to rule his group. He does a fantastic job, ruling by personality; he never beats anyone. Chico is dominant, but only because he is bigger and he beats people up, like Jack in *Lord of the Flies*." Again and again relationships seemed important; each chimp needed to remember an individual's character and its response to a situation in order to interact socially with it. Jim thought that if a chimp can't interpret the rules, including facial expression, then he can't get ahead and form alliances.

Jim decided to give the groups some ice lollies in my honor. They freeze fruit in buckets of water and throw them over the wire and the chimps go wild. The silverback grabbed the ice while the others sucked up to him, imploringly. We were up on a roof watching. Suddenly Jim told me to duck. A chimp, disappointed and iceless, started throwing rocks at us. Big ones. Very accurately.

We walked across to some young chimps being fostered by Sally, a mother chimp. Jeremy made her bottle-feed them; after all, a commitment is a commitment. Jim had noticed that she uses very few of her facial expressions with the babies compared with those shown when she was in a group. She does not, for instance, need fear. I asked Jim if he had worked with bonobo monkeys, supposedly the most intelligent of all nonhuman primates. Their faces are hairless and expressive, and they gaze at each other longer than other nonhuman primates. They make love facing each other. He had not, but took me to see a small, solitary, woolly monkey. There was only one other like her in captivity, in Holland. She came across and tried to touch Jim's hand through the glass. When he goes in she will grab him and hold on and it takes him half an hour to leave.

Jim had to leave now to sort out a replacement photocopier. They could not afford a new one and had the offer of a secondhand one, "I do monkeys, I don't do photocopiers." As he left I pointed out in the crowd a young boy in a Batman outfit. "I got this chimp who had been rescued in a Batman outfit and I just put him in the cage. When I went back next day and took off the outfit he peed like crazy. He had been trained not to soil the outfit. It must have been so painful, the poor kid."

I left Monkey World having learned that I could meet a chimp, indeed had met chimps with Jim, but that I could not get to know them—that required years. It was clear that facial expressions were not just social displays in nonhuman primates, but that relatedness and a relationship were necessary to interpret facial expression (and body language and vocalization) correctly in the context of the group, its relationships, and the personalities involved. Even in the strange hierarchical societies at Howlett's and Monkey World, an individual's immediate behavior was probably not enough to navigate one's way through relationships. I had glimpsed the societies in which primates live and the place of facial expression in social interaction and in the genesis of interpersonal relatedness. I wanted to look through external behavioral states and through facial displays to something beyond, to their intelligence and social groupings. I could not hope do that with another species in such a short time. So next I went to someone who had started to do this professionally before moving in another direction.

The Tavistock Institute, London

In the 1960s the major tranquilizers had just got going and a lot of patients with schizophrenia were being released into community care. Caroline Garland, an undergraduate from Cambridge, had gone to study experimental psychology in the United States. Living two blocks from a care center she went in and offered her services. She kept on going, so eventually they paid her. "That particular experience joined up with much of what I had been reading in English literature, with the oddities and the extremities of behavior. I came back to London, and started a doctorate in primate social behavior—which I did not finish—working with a colony of chimps at London Zoo and got to know them very well."

She is now a psychoanalyst. I was fascinated to know how she had moved from one discipline, studying primate behavior, "out there" and displayed to the world, to another, helping people with their emotional problems, much of which is never shown.

"An interesting question. I actually feel I may know what happens inside a chimpanzee when it is traumatized and I feel I do know what happens inside an adult human being. I have seen a lot of people following a catastrophic event, like seeing your mother murdered. Being captured by slave traders and seeing your family killed is what happens to young chimps. One upsetting case was a wife who could not have a baby. Her sailor husband had bought her a chimpanzee which was in a cot with a layerette blanket—everything as though for a baby. We called at 5:30 in the morning. The original scene when the baby was captured was replicated by us as we took away the chimp from the tragic couple."

I asked whether she felt that chimpanzees entered into relationships with each other. I asked if the more personal aspects of facial expression which humans may use are also present in chimpanzees, something that was less clear in the literature. I felt that a lot was going on at an affective level, without and before symbolic language.

"There is no conceptual information which can be transmitted without language, but there is a lot of emotional language which can be. When I got to know my young chimpanzees very well, because I was largely responsible for them, I realized after a while that they would soon know what sort of a mood I was in and they would respond to it with a sympathetic noise or they would be bouncy and lively and give an invitation to play. They have facial expression and body posture, vocalization, and hair erections; large combinations.

"The really expressive bit of a chimpanzee is its mouth. An enormous amount can be communicated by the degree of pout or the licking movement between a pout, which is an appeasing, beseeching expression of, "Please can I have?" and the grimace in which both rows of teeth are revealed, which is fear.

"In the smile the top lip is pulled down over the top teeth. It is usually a play face and indicates that whatever is to follow should not be taken amiss. If you bite or rampage with a fellow chimpanzee having made that face you are on reasonably safe ground. If you don't make that, then you are on uncertain ground. It is also an expression a chimpanzee can't help making. If you tickle a chimp it is obviously real and involuntary. Do chimpanzees smile at their own thoughts? I don't know. I do not think we can say what goes on inside a chimpanzee's mind in the same way we can in human beings. We can sit down and listen for hour after hour after hour [in analysis] and link up all the information we are getting from everywhere—except the face. We cannot do that with chimpanzees."

"But how much flexibility between facial display and behavior is there? If the links are not always fixed, then a chimp will need knowledge of others, will need relatedness and relationship, and an interpersonal memory. Do you need to know an individual to know what some more subtle expressions mean?"

"Absolutely. I think chimpanzees dream and when they dream they dream about other chimpanzees. If they do, then they may have some sort of version of what we call internal objects. Perhaps one way at getting at what you are asking is to ask, Are they capable of dissembling in the way human beings are? We can pretend to be feeling one thing but showing another."

This leads to Machiavellian intelligence, to deceit, which chimpanzees are supposed to be capable of. Burn and Whiten discuss Dewaal's observation of self correction in a chimp.[24] A male sitting with his back to a challenger showed a (fear) grin on hearing hooting. He quickly used his fingers to push his lips back over his teeth, a manipulation which occurred three times before the male turned to face his rival to bluff his way out of an attack. This suggested self-knowledge of facial display and its effect on others. Such work is still controversial. What is established, however, is that chimpanzees, but not most other nonhuman primates, have sufficient self-awareness to recognize the reflection of themselves in a mirror.[25]

I returned to Caroline's career change, and asked about the differences between chimpanzees and humans.

"I believed that the only way you can find out what is going on inside was by observing the externals and then watching for patterns and seeing what the consequences of those patterns were, so that after a while one could interpret expressions.

"I think ethologists miss out something very important and that is the subjective state. It is not that they are not interested in it. They just believe that you can only get at it through behavior. I remember how absolutely hair-raising it was to realize that I could communicate emotionally with individuals of another species, chimpanzees, so that one of them and I would look at each other and I would know what was happening in him and he would understand what was going on in me. One particular one, China, I thought of as a friend."

"Darwin talked of being drawn into facial observations. In exploring the essential aspects of being a person you can only do that if you take part in their world and engage in it."

"But that is what psychoanalysis is. I found primate ethology so difficult and eventually uncomfortable because I had to try to be an observer. I gave it up since I could no longer pretend that I was just an observer of what was going on. I was part of what was going on and I had strong feelings about it."

Caroline was concerned that we had not got far in discussing feeling states in nonhuman primates. For my part, however, her journey from ethology to analysis had revealed something which had been driving me, intuitively, from the outset. I could not understand the face, and understand the relation between expression and self, by observation and objectivity alone. To go further one had to enter a world of subjective witness, risking individual's reliability in talking of themselves and their personal experience.

Psychoanalysis used language to understand others, never looking at the face.[26] Perhaps facial contact required a more equal relationship than the controlled asymmetry between analyst and analysand. In trying to understand something of what the face represented I had to use language too, but language to describe what Freud had apparently ignored.

I was convinced by now that nonhuman primates' facial expressions were extraordinarily complex, being at times social displays and at other times emotional readouts, and that we needed some knowledge of, and relationship with, the individual to interpret all this accurately. Faces seemed to require individuality. This being the case, then any natural history of the face had to include the subjective narratives of those with facial problems and not just ethological observations and clinical studies from the outside.

Born Independent

6

I had learned that facial action was more than a predictor of behavior and a way to display and manipulate. But looking at primates had not allowed me to see precisely what the face did in humans. A dimension was still missing.

To display requires an observer, and with that the development of attention in others to facial display. Through facial action relationships between sender and recipient may evolve, with information flowing to and fro in a flexible and adaptable manner. Might this lead toward ideas that we might know what others are experiencing and feeling in part because of facial display?

Theory of Mind

In a famous experiment a young female gorilla in a zoo was presented with a problem. Opening the door to leave her cell required lifting a latch which was too high for her to reach. She had a box in her room and a human keeper. Solutions to the problem involved moving the box over to the door and climbing on it, dragging the human over and then climbing on him (using him as a box), and third, asking the human to open the latch. As she grew up over a year or so the gorilla solved the problem by using the three solutions successively.[1] In the third step, to make the man do what she wanted, the gorilla looked into his eyes, even though to check on his actions it would have been better to look at his arms. She was checking that the keeper was concentrating on her request and eye contact allowed shared attentional contact. The coordination of her desire and his action and its communication, and the interaction between two individuals, required shared attention, and the way this was produced was, in part, through gaze. Gaze, which in many primates species—if prolonged—represents threat, was here being used in a completely different way. It required two individuals to enter into a relationship. Gaze, either mutually toward an object, or mutually at each other, may be the first crucial condition for our leaving the world of display and facial reflexes.[2] Yet mutual attention is not sufficient: it will tell us where someone is looking, but the gorilla used gaze to influence another and to know something of the other's intentions.

In 1978 Premack and Woodruff described experiments with a chimpanzee called Sarah. She had learned a series of symbols which allowed them to show that she could predict and interpret human actions by use of mental states such as intention. They asked, in the title of their paper, "Does the chimpanzee have a theory of mind?" They explained, "An individual has a theory of mind if he imputes mental states to himself and others. A system of inferences of this kind is properly viewed as a theory because such states are not directly observable. . . "

Immediate behavior then, is not sufficient; clues about motive arise from things other than simple movement of the body.

The system may be used to make predictions about the behavior of others. As to the mental states the chimpanzee may infer, consider those inferred by our own species, for example, purpose, or intention, as well as knowledge, belief, doubt, guessing, pretending, liking and so forth. (p. 515)[3]

The authors' series of experiments asked the chimpanzee to view a videotape of a human trying to get at bananas out of reach, on the ceiling or outside a cage. The chimpanzee was given several photographs, one of which had a solution to the problem, for example, a stick to get the bananas, and asked to choose the correct one on the basis of understanding both the problem and the actor's purpose. She succeeded, though whether or not because she could make predictions about others, that is, had a "theory of mind," is still a matter of debate.[4]

Subsequently there has been a huge amount of work delineating aspects of mental development in terms of theory of mind. Wimmer and Perner used what has been called the Sally-Anne test.[5] They placed two boxes on a table before two children, "Sally" and "Anne." A marble was placed inside one box and so was hidden from view, though both children knew which box it was in. Then Sally was asked to go outside and the marble was put in the other box. When Sally came back in, Anne was asked which box Sally would look for her marble in. Success required Anne to understand that Sally would not know that the marble had been moved. Normal children passed this test by three to four years of age, so showing that they could put themselves in someone else's position.

The test was used by Simon Baron-Cohen, Alan Leslie, and Uta Frith, to show a defect in theory of mind in autistic children.[6] Many of the problems autistic persons have in social functioning may be traceable to an inability to read other people. The test, incidentally, was portrayed on stage in Peter Brook's play *The Man Who,* based on and inspired by Oliver Sacks's *Hat* book, to show something of the tragedy of autism.

The theory of mind has been enormously influential in a wide variety of disciplines, from developmental psychology to philosophy. Much of the work on theory of mind has involved *cognitive* "thinking" tests like the Sally-Anne test. But those inner mental states considered to be understood by theory of mind have ranged from beliefs, desires and intentions—states with a large thinking component—to much more "feeling," affective, or emotional ones. The theory requires self-knowledge of motivation and intent. It also has to explain how we are aware that others are feeling, desiring, intending what we think they are. How could these develop in a child? Some proponents of the theory accept that it is weak in explaining its origins. Leslie, for instance, has suggested that it is difficult to see how perceptual evidence could allow a child to invent the idea of unobservable mental states in others.[7] Perner suggested this empathy was possible by identifying another's inner emotional state as being similar to that which one is familiar with from one's own inner state.[8] Then that state can be projected as a theoretical construct onto the other to understand what is going on inside him or her.[9]

The origins of theory of mind were addressed recently by Simon Baron-Cohen in his book *Mindblindness*[10] (in which his ideas are explained by reference to autism). He suggests a model with four mechanisms: an intentionality detector, an eye direction detector, a shared attention mechanism, and lastly a theory-of-mind module. He unfurls the model with beautiful clarity and precision. There is, he suggests, innately within us, an "intentionality detector," which allows us to distinguish the motion of external objects, or animate beings, in terms of volitional mental states. This allows the crucial distinction to be made between whether motion was caused by an animate being or not. Then an infant can interpret this motion in terms of the mover's goal or desire.

Whereas the intentionality detector can operate through touch or sound as well as vision, the second mechanism, the eye direction detector, only works through vision. There are known to be potent neurophysiological mechanisms allowing an infant to detect another's eyes, to know if the eyes are looking at him or her or away, and then from this to know whether the gaze is mutual or not. The next step is to know that another's eyes are sharing in your view or ideas. The shared attention mechanism allows this by knowledge that the object of the infant's attention is shared, say, by her mother. This requires constant feedback that *my* object is *her* object of attention, so that both the object of attention and the mother's eyes must be monitored. Similarly, the three mechanisms must relate to one another, so that shared attention allows information about intentionality, for instance. The last step for Baron-Cohen is the development of a theory-of-mind mechanism, something that allows another to infer a full range of mental states so that behavior can be read in terms of the mental states of volition (desire and goal) and epistemy (pretending, thinking, imagining, etc.).[11]

Gaze direction is stressed as a way into another's mind. We do not only look at eyes. Birds and snakes, after all, can do this, reacting differently toward people according to their gaze direction. We go further than entering into mutual gazes: we interpret others' behavior in mentalistic ways that nonhuman primates do not. One way this quantum leap of mental development may have arisen is by increasing the amount of subtle mind states which in humans may be seen not just from the eyes but from the face as a whole. The face may be a necessary part of a development of a theory of mind.

Feelings of Soul

Baron-Cohen, in common with other cognitive psychologists, does not ignore emotion, but is able to say very little about its role, because in his view we are long way from having a good theory of it. He does accept that future theories of mind reading will have to admit it, "since it is self-evident that human beings are not 'cold' computational devices."

Others have attempted the difficult task of embedding emotion in the development of mind, so trying to untangle exactly what is "self-evident." Peter Hobson, professor at University College, London, and at the Tavistock Clinic, criticizes "theory of mind" at its very origin since for him it is hardly conceivable that a person can conceptualize his own mental states as a precondition to ascribing similar states to others.[12]

Hobson's arguments are complex, not least because he attempts to place our awareness of others, and their motives, in a domain beyond the cognitive area, in which the theory of mind has been expressed, and into areas of feeling and emotion which are on the boundaries of scientific experimentation. He suggests that the difficulties in calibrating a mental state as being the same in one individual as in another can be avoided if there are observable criteria for some mental states. These must also be public for agreement between people about what constitute particular subjective experiences. Something like anger must exist not only as a subjective inner state but must also be observable in facial, gestural, and vocal expression. If so, then the feeling state "anger" is not understood by constructing a theory of mind but is directly observed in others and oneself.

Hobson agrees that once one has acquired the notion of persons with a subjective mental life, one can infer things on the basis of analogy from one's own case. The problem is in whether the ascribing of mental life to others can *arise* through reasoning by analogy or through introspection or inference. He suggests that initially we do not perceive others as objects into which we learn to place minds, like engines in cars.

It is not the case that the concept of "persons" is somehow derivative from some more primitive notions of "bodies" on the one hand and "minds" on the other. Instead, the apprehension of person-related "meanings" is a primary form of perception, and the concept of "persons" is more fundamental than either the concept of "bodies" or the concept of "minds." (p. 185)[12]

In their original paper Premack and Woodruff gave examples of the cognitive states of purpose and intents: knowledge and thinking. Later, others included emotion—and indeed Perner chose such a "feeling" example to explain how theories of mind may be constructed. For Hobson these emotional states are first felt and then related to self and to others, and where they are felt and expressed is to a major degree the face.

Consider a mother and child in the first few days and weeks after birth. Daniel Stern has described the choreography of faces, voices, and bodily movements that goes on between the mother and the newborn child as the very beginnings of the infant's knowledge of the world.[13, 14] This knowledge begins with relatedness between mother and baby, and possibly begins before thought and before language. Though not the sole form of communication, eye contact and facial expressions are a most important part of a child's realization of the category of others. Before gesture, before eloquent vocalization, the face is the essence of the individual and this is why a baby's use of the face is so advanced in comparison to her ability to move other body parts effectively. Try, if you can, to imagine a young baby without any ability to move his or her face.

For Hobson the very core of what a baby needs and does, what we all need and do, is relate to others. It is driven not by a need to construct theories of others' minds but by a basic, essential requirement to feel the comforts of others, to be with someone in the world, to be in relation-ship to another, to have oneself reflected in another. This is not learned but given—innate, within us all; with and before the cognitive is the emotional. And the other made manifest is seen first, and most perhaps, in the face.

The Color of Hair

Some of the most devastating effects of absence or loss of facial anima-tion have been shown to be on social interaction, as will be seen in later chapters. But there are also some conditions in which abnormal social interaction is considered a primary problem. Many of the differing ideas about cognitive development, interpersonal relatedness, and the theory of mind have been developed in relation to a single clinical condition, autism.

Described independently by Leo Kanner[15] in 1943 and by Hans Asperger[16] in 1944, the clinical features of autism include impaired social development, delayed and deviant language, and insistence on sameness. There are many pictures of autism, however, from the self-mutilating institutionalized child, to persons with savant skills in art and music. Two beautiful accounts concerning an autistic artist and a famous "Anthropologist on Mars" are to be found in Oliver Sacks's book of that title.[17] Sacks makes the point that "No two people with autism are the same; its precise form or expression is different in every case. . . . while a single glance may suffice for clinical diagnosis, if we hope to understand the autistic individual, nothing less than a total biography will do."

Fortunately, such biographies and occasional autobiographies have appeared to allow this for a few individuals.[18] Though Kanner and Asperger wrote at the same time, their emphases were slightly different. This has led to a division of affected individuals into one of two categories: *autism* or *Asperger syndrome,* with the former considered more severely affected and the latter higher-functioning. The cause of the difference between these two groups remains unclear. For Sacks, "the ultimate difference, perhaps, is this: people with Asperger syndrome can tell us of their experiences, their inner feelings and states, whereas those with classical autism cannot."[19]

What has fascinated and frustrated those trying to understand, and help, those "with" autism has been how difficult it is to reach these children. They have an asocial aspect, apparently unable to relate to other people, as though "born independent,"[20] a phrase which sums up their solitariness but not their vulnerability. Indeed Kanner entitled his original paper, "Autistic Disturbances of Affective Contact," highlighting, right at the beginning, their difficulties in entering and maintaining relationships with other people. Asperger, in describing the population he saw, wrote,

When we talk to someone we do not only "answer" with words, but we "answer" with our look, our tone of voice and the whole expressive play of face and hands. A large part of social relationships is conducted through eye gaze, but such relationships are of no interest to the autistic child. Therefore the child does not generally bother to look at the person who is speaking . . .

. . . autistic children have a paucity of facial and gestural expression. In ordinary two-way interaction they are unable to act as a proper counterpart to their opposite number, and hence they have no use for facial expression as a contact-creating device.

I set out to try to understand if social relationships were truly of no interest to autistic persons. Was it really that they did not bother to look at the person speaking, and so had no use for facial expression, as some had suggested,[21] or did they bother so much that they had to avoid eye contact? How did their condition and their "facial avoidance" relate to one another, and what could we learn from autistic subjects about the use of the face in ourselves as *the* representation of the other.

The lack of relatedness between autistic people and others is reflected in our inability to relate to them, and hence in our difficulties in understanding; it is at the core of the problem. What this "lack" is has been explained by the cognitive school as being in "theory of mind," and in the affective, emotional relatedness between people. In contrast Delacato[22] proposed that the problem with autistic children might be an inability to decipher incoming information. Some were hypersensitive to sound, or to light or touch, whereas others were almost oblivious to such sensations. Either way sensations and perceptions were so scrambled that they were unintelligible; sounds or images so were fuzzy or unformed that they were meaningless, and not just meaningless, but frightening and overwhelming. Delacato suggested that autistic persons live in a fog, or nightmare, unable to make sense, to have sense, of what is happening around them or to them.

It is difficult to imagine living in such a world, and many—most—autistic persons are unable to communicate it. So the experiences of autistic subjects who have been able to communicate their experience have been especially important. Temple Grandin certainly wrote of both sensory overload and of being insensitive.[23]

Intensively preoccupied with the movement of the spinning coin or lid, I saw nothing or heard nothing. People around me were transparent. And no sound intruded . . . Even a sudden loud noise didn't startle me from my world.

But when I was in the world of people, I was extremely sensitive to noises . . . a forty minute trip on a ferry—exciting and adventurous to Mother and my younger sisters and brothers—was a nightmare of sound to me, violating my ears and very soul.

Relatedness, theory of mind, overload, these theories have allowed much insight into autism, though how the consequences of each determine the others and interact have scarcely begun to be addressed. Whichever might hold, a recurring problem for autistic persons in their lack of relatedness is a difficulty in that most simple and yet important aspect of reducing the distance between people, namely, looking at the face.

There do seem to be differences for people with autism between looking at animals and humans, and particularly in looking at others' faces. That there is such a specific problem suggests an *active avoidance* rather than a "not bothering" with facial contact, and implies therefore that autistic individuals do have some concept of the face that is problematic. Maybe they have some realization that faces, in some way, are an entry point to others and to the autistic person themselves. And without some realization of mind, both one's own and others, social understanding and communication are scarcely possible.[24]

The problems with the face and gaze of persons with autism have been approached by careful experimentation: some observers consider that difficulties in reciprocal gaze and eye contact are among the most striking manifestations of autism.[25] Such work sits uneasily with other experiments showing quite clearly that autistic children can recognize photographs of emotions like "happy" and "sad" as well as age- and IQ-matched children.[26] Baron-Cohen et al.[27] were more probing. They argued that, since simple "sad-happy" emotional recognition was apparently normal in autism, the deficit could not be a general one in understanding affect. In contrast, if understanding surprise was more difficult for autistic children, it might be because surprise—that something unusual or unpredictable had happened—needed a cognitive component. That "cognitive emotion" recognition was abnormal in autism could then be explained by a lack of theory of mind. Without wishing to descend into definitions (is a "cognitive" emotion, like surprise or shock, an emotion at all?), work with autistic subjects and their use of the face has shown deficits in shared attention, gaze behavior, and in complex, but not in simple, emotion recognition. This work has been most revealing about some of the problems of autistic people, but does not allow for a full understanding of the *reasons* for those problems.

Caroline Garland concluded that to study internal states subjective experience had to be admitted, leading her from ethology to an understanding of humans' minds via psychoanalysis. In asking questions about the face and autistic persons' difficulties with facial expression, I too had to ask about subjective experience, if indeed that existed with autism. By asking about problems with the face and facial expressivity, I reasoned, might one be led to some semblance of understanding of mind in autism, or would the problem with mind and affect, and overload, preclude such introspection?

Until recently, personal witness from Asperger and particularly autistic persons have been absent. Now, slowly, reports are emerging, spilling out astonishing stories, streams of experience, even if they might not be—could not be—Joycean streams of consciousness. But in the present context my primary interest was not in the owned experience of autism but with the difficulties that autistic persons have with looking at people, at what it is about the face which is so perplexing. In asking about less than a whole life I was asking them to *reorder* their experience in a way I had directed, possibly a far more difficult task than an autobiography.

Through a colleague I went to see David, a man in his late teens, who has Asperger syndrome. He is "high functioning," for he lives alone, although he has had difficulty in keeping jobs. As we chatted, with his parents present, the only suggestion of a problem was a slight slowness and deliberation. He was only diagnosed at age sixteen when his mother remarried and her new husband realized that something was seriously amiss. David's early years at school had been without achievement—mostly he remembered the bullying, when his "differences" from the others were so cruelly exposed, though never explained.[28] I asked how he recognized and tried to understand people. "I do it by voice, or look—mostly voice. I know what someone else is thinking or feeling by somewhere between an educated guess and by looking at the face and how they are sitting. There are a couple of friends that I can tell what they are thinking by looking at them 'cos their body language is so strong."[29]

Here it is unlikely that the friends' body language was any stronger than others,' so that for David knowing the person helped understand them. I asked the big theory-of-mind question. "Can you put yourself in someone else's shoes, try to know what it is like to be that person?"

"Sometimes, but very often, no."[30]

"When I see your mother smiling I don't think, 'She's smiling,' I think she is happy (processing beyond what is seen, to its significance). When you see someone smiling—"

"It means I don't feel happy for them, though they may feel happy in themselves. You can smile and yet feel real sad inside. In the street I am a naturally nosy person. I like to know what kind of person is on the inside and outside. I use color of hair, length of stride of walk, whether they have got their arms crossed. If it's red hair, that can change personality. A big stride indicates a strong person; the color of clothes also helps. This is all from a book I read recently."[31]

"Everything used except the face—"

"I look at faces, wanting to know if the stare is prolonged, then it feels like it is a threat. So in the second or two you have got to look at a person you are making judgments about yourself. When they look at me, they may be making the same decisions that I would be making about them."

So for David, at least, others do make judgments too, do have minds. Note also that he has a few friends he can know about; his problem has imposed an intimacy somewhat like that found in the blind subjects. He continued,

"I think if you determine how someone's character is based, you've got more indication how they will behave. You can guess people's emotional state from their face, but you can't really know much about their personality."

I agreed completely. David seemed to have worked out some aspects of others not apparent from my reading.

"One of the things that does concern me is that I might not feel[32] worried or anything that I should be feeling, and my mum will ask me how I feel, and I will say it doesn't bother me.[33]

In much of what David had said his problems stemmed from an inability to concentrate on all that was going on, from an overload. In a pub washing up he was fine, but when asked to fetch something from another room he lost concentration, went "off-line." He described how he had to concentrate the whole time in order to function in the world. I once wrote a book about a man, a friend, who had lost all sense of touch and joint and movement sense.[34] The only way he could learn to move again was by looking at his body and by *thinking,* the whole time, all day, each day, about movement. We attempted to describe the mental concentration involved as a daily marathon. David seemed to be living in a similar world but for different reasons, a daily marathon to attend in order to make any sense of the world.[35] I said that most of us could go through a day without having to concentrate at all.[36] "I can't do that.

In a builder's I would be sweeping the yard[37] and I would have to serve a customer,[38] and then I would forget what I was doing. I would get bollocked, but I had forgotten what I was doing."

This thoughtless and pointless punishment would have been incomprehensible to David and so reinforced his disorientation. I asked about others being happy, or sad or worried. Could he take them in?

"In other people? No. If my mother is sad or happy or angry, then probably, but others . . . With her I might know it but I don't feel it."[39]

"So how do you know what she is feeling?"

"I look in her face. I have always known that happiness is shown on the face."

By rote learning, I presumed, which allowed recognition of the simple expressions but not the more complex ones. I continued, "But when I see someone happy it tends to make me join their expression and be the same."

"It doesn't happen with me. I won't laugh unless it is funny. It is not funny if I do not laugh."[40]

For David there was no social laughter, no pretense (a little like David Blunkett, who complained of blind people not being taught to smile socially). I said that when we look at others we can't help but to begin to feel similar things, be influenced by others.

"I do not feel that."

Some autistic persons will echo the expressions and actions of others. But they do not feel what they are expressing or caricaturing.[41] I thought of Wittgenstein who had wondered whether a smile that did not make him smile could be a real smile at all. But he had not wondered what sort of existence was possible if the invitations and seductions in facial expression could not be experienced by an observer.[42] For David, it was clear. He could recognize simple rote-learned emotions on the face, but could not process complex ones,[43] as predicted by theory-of-mind experiments. But recognition of emotion in someone else had no power to move him; he could not empathize with them and so there was little capacity to relate or engage with another.

The psychological theories seemed here to be side by side, complementary in looking at different aspects of the same fragmented "personality" with which people with Asperger's may exist. Did either single explanation explain the problem, or could it be that the inability arose because of problems of sensory overload, leading to sensations being confused and uninterpretable? Whatever explanation, or combination of explanations, was correct, the difficulties in looking at faces were at its core. By exploring autism and the face I became convinced one could understand something of what the face meant in us "normal" nonautistic persons despite autistic subjects' many and obvious problems both in perception and in its analysis and communication.

I was very conscious that David had not and could not have considered such matters. He had agreed to see me with his parents, and for that I was very grateful. But I felt that to go further might be possible only with someone with autism who had *automatically* expressed some interest in such matters. I turned to an autistic savant writer who has written on the subject, Donna Williams. Reading my interview with David she had replied,

Face is a mistrusted system upon which expectation is weighed with little hope of meeting it. To see others seeking to use a system that doesn't work is to see sharply one's own alien-ness . . . To coordinate socially look and smile requires too much processing, accessing and monitoring of both external and internal stimuli for it to be successful.

If look and smile were too much in an immediate context, then her books had shown her astonishing gifts at analysis through writing. I wrote asking her about the face, slightly fearing what might be her reply to yet another request for information.

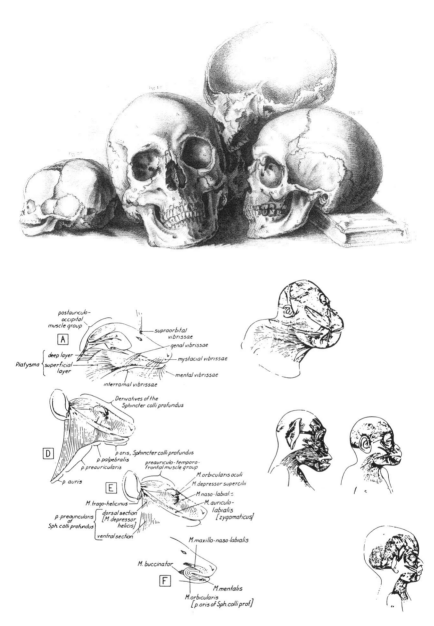

Figure 1   Skull of a man fully grown, presented in a front view and in profile, a section of the cranium, and skull of a child. (From Sir Charles Bell, *Essays on the Anatomy and Philosophy of Expression*, 2nd ed. London: John Murray, 1824.)

Figure 2   Schema of primate ground plan of the superficial facial musculature. (*left*) A shows the platysma muscle and its derivatives in "primitive primates." D. The sphincter colli muscle and its derivatives. (*right*) The superficial facial musculature of the three great anthropoid apes, orangutan, chimpanzee, and gorilla, and a new-born child. (From Huber, In *The Evolution of Facial Expression: Two Accounts*, New York: Arno Press, 1972.)

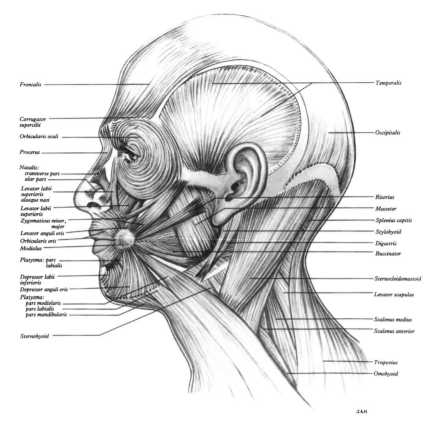

Frontalis

Corrugator supercilii

Orbicularis oculi

Procerus

Nasalis:
  transverse part
  alar part

Levator labii superioris alaeque nasi

Levator labii superioris

Zygomaticus minor, major

Levator anguli oris

Orbicularis oris

Modiolus

Platysma: pars labialis

Depressor labii inferioris

Depressor anguli oris

Platysma:
  pars modiolaris
  pars labialis
  pars mandibularis

Sternohyoid

Temporalis

Occipitalis

Risorius

Masseter

Splenius capitis

Stylohyoid

Digastric

Buccinator

Sternocleidomastoid

Levator scapulae

Scalenus medius

Scalenus anterior

Trapezius

Omohyoid

J.A.H.

Figure 3   Dissection of a face. Note the prominence given to the modiolus, which was often ignored in earlier anatomical drawings. Dissection of the face allows a view of the underlying muscles. It is a poor way of looking at facial anatomy and function, however, since many muscles of facial expression are embedded in the skin and their structure cannot be shown. (From *Gray's Anatomy*, 34th ed., 1995. Reprinted with permission of Churchill Livingstone.)

Figure 4   (*opposite, top*) Photographic plate of electrically induced expression of joy. Duchenne used a seductive wanton, a narcissistic actor, an opium addict who died two days after the experiment and, most frequently, this man in his stimulation experiments. The man he described as being "an old toothless man, with a thin face, whose features, without being absolutely ugly, approached ordinary triviality and whose facial expression was in perfect agreement with his inoffensive character and his restricted intelligence." Duchenne's reasons for choosing him were revealing and uplifting: "I have preferred this coarse face to one of noble, beautiful features . . . because I wanted to prove that, despite defects of shape and lack of plastic beauty, every human face can become spiritually beautiful through the accurate rendering of emotions." The man also had reduced sensation over the face, an advantage when having it connected to a "double current volta-faradic apparatus." We are led to believe that he felt no pain when the muscles of the face were stimulated to produce this expression of joy. (From Duchenne du Boulogne, op. cit.)

Figure 5   (*opposite, bottom*) Photographic plate of electrically induced expression of pain. (From Duchenne du Boulogne, op. cit.)

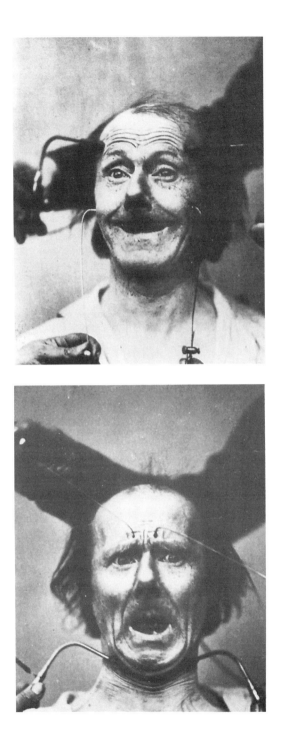

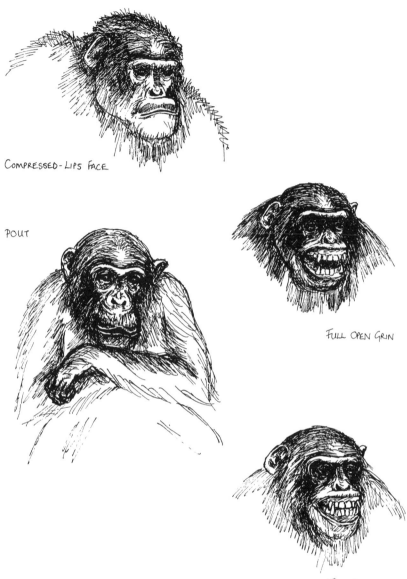

COMPRESSED-LIPS FACE

POUT

FULL OPEN GRIN

FULL CLOSED GRIN

Figure 6   Four typical facial expressions in chimpanzees. Compressed-lips face: display. Pout: distress. Full open grin and full closed grin: different levels of fear/excitement. Drawn by Rosalind Alp while undertaking field work in Sierre Leone. (Courtesy of the artist.)

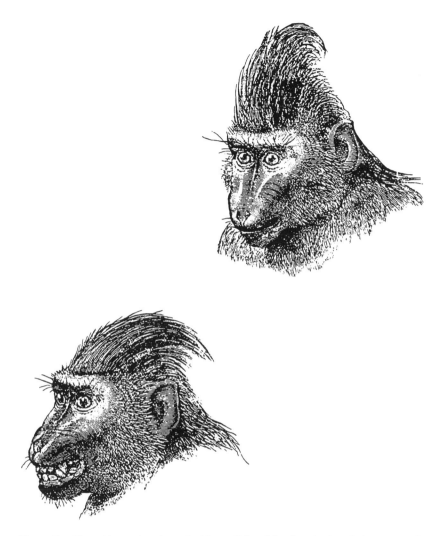

Figure 7 *Cynopithecus niger*, in a placid condition (*above*) and when being caressed (*below*). Drawn from life by Mr. Wolf. (From Charles Darwin, *The Expression of the Emotions in Man and Animals*. Reprint Chicago: University of Chicago Press, 1965.)

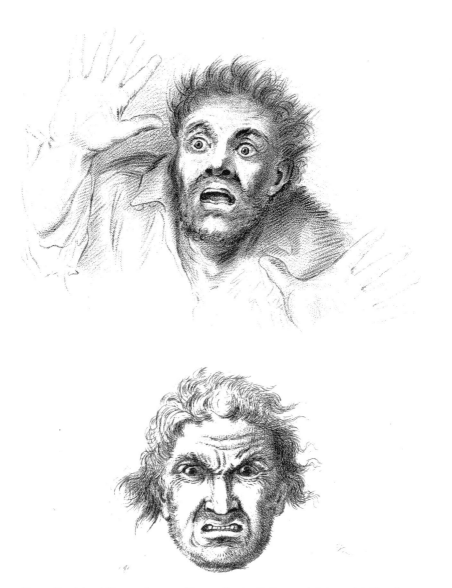

Figure 8   (*above*) Fear and anger. (From Charles Bell, op. cit.) (*opposite*) Happiness, fear, and anger. Posed expressions in a manner similar to those used by Ekman and colleagues. Note the similarity to Bell's drawings. The expressions are rather extreme but chosen to be unambiguous. (Reproduced with permission from D. Keltner and B. N. Buswell, "Evidence for the Distinctness of Embarrassment, Shame, and Guilt," *Cognition and Emotion* 10[1996]: 155–171.)

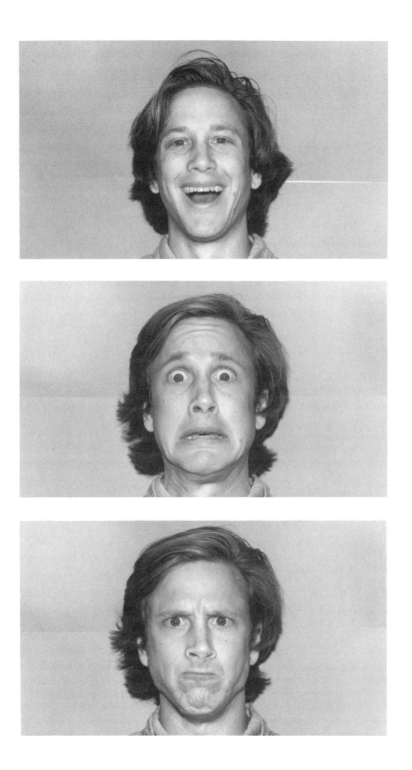

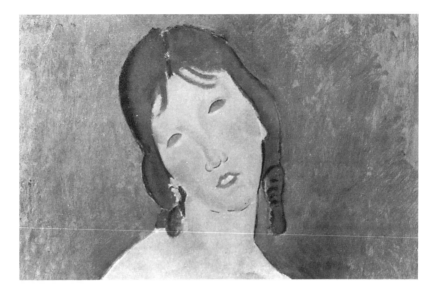

Figure 9   *The Little Milkmaid,* detail, by Amedeo Modigliani, c.1918. The face, with its rather blank wrinkleless expression and slack mouth, has a similarity to some of those with Möbius syndrome. Modigliani used blank pupils for artistic effect in several portraits, and I know of no evidence that he saw someone with Möbius. Collection of Mr. George Friedland, Philadelphia, Pennsylvania. (From Gaston Diehl, *Modigliani,* New York: Crown Publishers, 1969.)

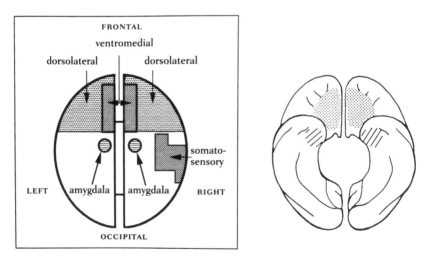

Figure 10   (*left*) Diagram representing the regions damage to which compromises aspects of reasoning and processing of emotion. (*right*) Diagram showing the amygdala (hatched), and the orbitofrontal cortex (dotted), areas thought to be involved in the theory-of-mind mechanism. (Left panel reprinted by permission of the Putnam Publishing Group from *Descartes' Error* by Antonio R. Damasio, M.D. Copyright © 1994 by Antonio R. Damasio, M.D. Right panel from L. Brothers, "The Social Brain," *Concepts in Neuroscience* 1[1990]: 27–51.)

Like a Ball Off a Wall

7

Donna Williams has thus far written two books on her life, *Nobody Nowhere*[1] and *Somebody Somewhere*.[2] She has laid bare her personal experience of living as an autistic person, which for her has been a most astonishingly rich emotional journey. In the previous chapter I wrote that I was not concerned with portraying a whole life, for that might be an imposition or threat; her books have done this, in the most powerful and extraordinary detail.

She was born in Australia, in the 1960s, and lived her early years in her own world, struggling for any semblance of understanding of what was going on. Though bright, she ended up in a special school and was tested for deafness at around age seven because of her lack of responsiveness to sounds and voices. She was not, however, slow at learning and came second in her primary school leaving exams. But after this her teens were spent dropping out of one school after another, alternately being disruptive and picked on. At fifteen she left for a succession of jobs, as a sewing machinist in a fur coat company and as a shop assistant. The first boy she met she went to live with, much to his surprise. He beat her and abused her. There followed a series of flats and jobs and boys.

At the age of eighteen she decided that she wanted to go back to school. Her favorite subject was psychology and she passed the year with sufficient marks to go to university where she entered a school of social studies. She was able to make friends with one or two men who did not let her down, and after three years passed her finals well enough to be accepted for a thesis. After that she drifted again, choosing the wrong men, living for a while in a garage and finding work in a theatrical shop, fascinated by the masks and wigs. She did some traveling and met and befriended a man "like her" on a train who turned out to have a form of autism. She left for England, found a job as a secretary, then fell into writing her story. She also discovered for the first time that she was autistic, something she greeted with excitement and relief to have found a name for her experience.

She went back to Australia and entered a long series of meetings and correspondence with a psychiatrist or psychologist who did much to help her to understand herself. At this time she also trained to be a primary schoolteacher and finished that course successfully before a return visit to England and then America, this time to see the publishers of her first book. After a time back in Australia she left for England for good, initially promoting the book. She found a quiet cottage in the country, "feeling content." One day she crossed the road to a piano shop and met a quiet willowy figure, Ian, who was, again, "like her." The rest of her second book is given over to Ian and their beautifully moving love story. They are now married and live in quiet green rolling country close to the sea in the west of the United Kingdom.

Such bare facts do not begin to explore the emotional colors of her life, nor do they convey the tone of her experiences; these are only evident from her writings. The books are revelatory in allowing us to see Donna's journey from having little or no insight into her existence, to her discovery of her own unique world and its relation to others. Her language throughout is not that of an unemotional, unengaged person, but of quite the reverse, of a most gifted person trying to *consciously* [3] express and feel and belong to a world of experience she was overwhelmed by—yet dependent on for her existence. Sounds, lights, patterns, people, all were so overwhelming *in their sense of other* that they threatened and prevented what little sense of "self" that she could hold onto. Autism for her, then, means an almost unimaginable sensory fluctuating and processing problem and overload, which made it difficult for her to make sense of her world, or herself, at all. But her problems are not confined to sensory overload. They include a huge emotional component; toward the end of her first book she gives her opinion that,

Human beings are made up of three systems which in the normal person are reasonably integrated: mind, body and emotions. In some people one of these is at fault and makes complete integration impossible . . .

Retardation is an example where the mental or intellectual mechanism has broken down, constraining normal expression of one's self through an otherwise healthy body and emotions. Spasticity's a case where the body function is faulty and traps and constrains the expression of a healthy mind and emotions.

I believe that autism is the case where some sort of mechanism which controls emotion does not function properly, leaving an otherwise relatively normal mind unable to express itself with a depth that it otherwise is capable of. (pp. 181–182)

Though sensory overload is a perceived problem, she sees her autism as primarily an emotional problem.

Most of us accept unthinkingly that we live in a body, with a sense of that body as a whole and as the place where our mind lives, and can direct attention at will, to ourselves, to others, to any aspect of the world or of our thoughts. For Donna Williams, being "monotrack," not even these certainties existed. As a child, she wrote, she would stare into a mirror communing with the person she saw, giving her a name, trying to reach her.[4] Toward the end of her second book, writing of a time when she was in her twenties, she described the experience of touching her hand against her leg and consciously experiencing for the first time the two as connected, of her body as a whole,

My hand was placed randomly on my leg. Suddenly I became aware of inner feeling in both my hand and my leg at the same time. "I can feel my leg," I shouted in fear. I can feel my hand *and* my leg!" . . . I moved my hand to my arm and fearfully whispered, "I've got an arm." I felt it not on my hand from the outside, as usual, but from the inside. "Arm" was more than a texture; it was an inner sense . . .

My hands went up to my face. My face was there from the inside. My body was more than just a series of textures that my hands knew, an image my eyes saw . . .

My grasp on a direct . . . inner experience of whole life would probably always be transient, but my emotions and my thoughts and the connections between the two would be a consistent thread to hold it all together. (pp. 229–230)

While reading her books I kept returning to her problems in relations with others and the way in which, even from her early childhood when her ability to find any sense or reason in her world was severely limited, the face still played some role in defining people and so represented both threat and hope. She wrote that as a child she "avoided looking into other people's eyes, but could look into those of young baby brother." Once her father's eyes seemed to be crying out to reach her.

She learned to behave in a way that allowed her to function, painting a smile across her face, trying "to impersonate my version of happy." Smiling was not a pretense but a necessary way of existing.[5] At home there was one person she could look at,[6] her reflection in a mirror. "At home I would still spend hours in front of the mirror, staring into my own eyes and whispering my name . . . frightened at losing my ability to feel myself." She gave her mirror image a name, not her name but someone she had met in a park.[7] "Carol came in through the mirror . . . [she] looked just like me, but the look in her eyes betrayed her identity. I began to talk to her, and she copied me. I was angry . . . I began to whisper to her, putting my face very close to hers and wondering why she didn't turn to hear." She tried to join Carol, or Alice, in the mirror, but found she could not and remained alone. Later she wrote of "a horrified look on the boss' face." Her perception of emotion was beyond the simple. Perhaps she had some idea or "factual knowledge" of others' minds as well as faces. "I looked up at Mary, who seemed to have tears in her eyes. I was touched that she was able to feel emotion for my words in a way I had never been able to. I said nothing."[8]

She did not, however, feel that she resided in her body. "He kissed me—or perhaps I should say that he kissed my face, as I wasn't in it at the time." In reaching out she was looking for relatedness and yet shrinking from it. When she fell in love, "We both found it extremely difficult to look into each others' eyes, and when we did it was again the frightening feeling of losing oneself." To become too close was to be overwhelmed by the "otherness" of that person and to risk losing all connection to the fragile sense of "self." Time and time again she writes of how she would paint on a smile learned from a TV soap to hide from others her true feelings about the fragmented and very different view of the world that the autism allowed. Then as a teenager she found truth on her face when she ended a relationship, and her expression was connected to her feelings. "I felt the happiest I had for years, and for once it was reflected in the expression on my face, which was peaceful." Sometime after, "to love" was not to run but to involve and include relatedness. "He kissed me for the first time. I broke into tears. It was the first time in my life I had really "been there" whilst I had been kissed." Slowly the sharing of attention was not just seen as a threat, though the face and its gaze continued to represent an overwhelming presence of another.[9] "He was looking deeply into my eyes. I kept looking away. Yet, with each challenging remark, I would glare at him and he would capture me again. I had finally held Julian's stare and tried not to run away."

At the end of her first book she looked back at photos and saw how she had avoided looking at others, both to protect her self and to reduce information overload.

Looking back at the photos, I had recognised three ways in which I had avoided looking at people. One was to look straight through what was in front of me. Another was to look away at something else. The third was to stare blankly ahead with one eye and turn the other one inwards . . . blurring whatever view I had. (p. 173)

Having begun to reduce information overload she had developed sufficient concept of her self that she could gaze, look, and attempt to engage with others and in particular with a young autistic girl, and to understand the power of her gaze,[10]

Anne's crossed eyes were frozen in a dead stare, and she became silent between sobs. I took her hand and made her tap her own arm as I had, the tune and the rhythm and the tapping held totally constant.

I heard a soft but audible rhythm coming from outside me. Anne was making the tune herself in her throat, and I slowly dropped notes of my humming and, as I expected, she filled them in as though they were and had been her own. Slowly I dropped out more and more of them until she was doing not only the rhythm in her throat but carrying the tune as she tapped herself in time. Then, for a few frozen fifteen seconds, in that torchlit dark room she completely uncrossed her eyes for the first time since I'd met her and looked directly into my face as she tapped and hummed. (p. 177)

She had used her face, her gaze, her shared attention, to relate.

In her second book she continues her reflections on her motives, about her own mind, and those of others. The connection, or lack of connection, between these aspects and her face is immediate. "Autism had been there before thought . . . Autism had been there before sound . . . Autism had been there before I'd learned how to use my own muscles, so that every facial expression or pose was a cartoon reflection of those around me. Nothing was connected to self."[11]

She relates seeing truth and facade on the faces of others, both those unaffected and other autistic people,

Robbie's face was as dead and bland as a McDonald's as he ambled into the small room. For an instant on his way back out I had caught him smiling as he glanced momentarily for the first time at one of the objects he had been given . . . he had smiled as he glanced just before the curtains were drawn again across his face . . . I had seen Robbie in there . . . If only for an instant he had dared to have a self. (p. 21)

On several occasions she discusses meeting other autistic persons and often self seems to have been revealed through the face. Yet still, for most of the time, there was no clear relation between the face she showed the world and what she felt. Someone asked her,

"Smile, will you? Just be happy," a mechanical, production line look-alike smile appearing on my own face . . . "That's better." I burned with the injustice of having been taught to put a smile on the face of hatred . . . Facial expression had everything to do with learning to perform and nothing to do with feelings. Something inside me now told me this was wrong. (p. 54)

Despite this increasing understanding the awful sensory confusion and overload had not gone away and continued to threaten her constantly, and in this we may see one of the problems with the face—there was simply too much information to decode. Once she asked, "Can you take the dancing out of your voice [intonation] and not pull faces [facial expression]?" After discussing these things—through letters—with an educational psychologist she was beginning to see that "pulling faces" did *do* something. She writes of seeing emotion and facial expression together in a child.

I watched the ease with which she hugged her parents. I watched the expression on her face . . . What she did was not just for image, for acceptance. It was not out of insecurity to make sure they would still like her. There was something happening for her that affected not her expression but the change in her expression. What she did had come from feelings, and the change in her expression seemed like a dialogue between her and her parents.

She had felt something, acted upon it, gotten feedback, and expressed the way this changed or built upon her feelings. (pp. 132–133)

With professional help she could now see it, recognize it, recognize a conversation, and reflect upon it. "I was moved by what I saw. I could understand it and could begin to understand the difference between what I had known and what this girl had . . . "

Her own personal testament had opened her emotional world of autism, showing her own inner life to be truncated, disorganized,[12] but, primarily, necessarily and richly, emotional. Yet she had been unable to calibrate any of this by attention to others, by conscious and voluntary social referencing, nor by analysis of her own responses.[13] Part of the way in which she had begun to know of our world seemed to include observation of the face and facial expression. A repeated theme was that face represented personhood and feelings. Her journey to learn this was among the greatest of journeys I had read.

I wrote to her, explaining my interest. We corresponded, with me sending my stupid questions and half-understandings of her burning bright prose, and her putting me right when I had misunderstood, bluntly. ("Bullshit," she wrote once, and I agreed.) She said she would prefer not to meet, so I sent her ten pages of my ideas about the face and autism, and about my understanding of her books. I did not know whether I had been unfair to ask so much of her. Then one Easter Saturday, as we were entertaining a family to tea, the phone rang. It was Donna saying that she might meet me after all, and that she would send a fax to my home. I rushed to receive it, thinking it would be about dates, conditions, and addresses. In part it was, but it also contained her replies to my questions about her problems with faces. The fax machine whirred on and on, and as I read I became more and more astonished.

I had asked first why faces were so difficult and how she had been able to look into her brother's eyes but not into those of others,

My difficulties in looking at faces were a) to stand looking, b) to comprehend what I saw.

A. TO STAND LOOKING.
These were based on several things.
  1. Fear based on learning that looking would cause people to attempt to engage me in interaction—the fear of this was for three reasons in turn.
    (1) Such interaction would engulf my selfhood in a flood of "other."
    (2) Such interaction would evoke body sensation caused by intense emotion that would be beyond my ability to process, and therefore be confusing and frightening, and also be physically intolerable. These physical effects look and probably feel similar to what is seen when a junkie is in the grip of withdrawal tremors and intense muscle contraction, all combined with an intense feeling of being totally out of control.

For William James the emotion was its bodily expression. Here she made a distinction between the feeling and something taking place "out there" in a body. There is therefore some awareness of an implicit self and of body. We are all afraid of "letting go" of our emotions (see chapters 7 and 8). In autism, with fewer controls over feelings, the dangers are evidently far, far greater.

> (3) Such interaction would generally be only inconsistently comprehensible and would soon cause information overload after a few minutes and be poured down onto to me with a total absence of my own social interest or want.

1A. NOT BEING ABLE TO STAND LOOKING.
> Not being able to stand looking was because I could see that people were not true to their self and that made them scary. I could see if they were true to themselves or not because the eyes had no correlation to the expression of the rest of the face, and I was struck fiercely by the impact of this asymmetry. Its implications were that these people were somehow dangerous because their real self was not accessible. The difference between me and the others was that I was aware of this shift and did not confuse it with selfhood.
>
> It is when I see dead eyes in an animated face that I know the person is soul dead or at least disconnected. When I see alive eyes in a dead face I know the person is trapped in there and having trouble connecting with expression or daring to. When I looked in my brother's eyes, I saw someone like "me." What I mean by this is that I saw the same pattern of disconnection—a face contorted by grimace with non-smiling but alive eyes, a face with alive eyes but no connection to the face.
>
> I did not empathize with what the face was expressing but with the system that the facial disconnections spoke of. When I searched in my own eyes, [when looking in a mirror for hours on end] I did not look at my face, I searched for connectedness between soul and expression through body—most of the time I found none, except in my eyes. Sometimes I saw dead eyes in an animated face, sometimes I saw alive eyes in a disconnected face.

Here once more she is suggesting that she did have a concept of self,[14] and of others, but that perhaps the information overload resulted in processing problems that prevented her from simultaneously attending to both, or realizing herself in relation to others fully. The face, even her own face, was too complex for her to use and she looked instead at posture. Posture may in fact be easier to decode and it is no surprise, therefore, that animals and nonhuman primates use it, nor that Temple Grandin (an eminent designer of animal houses and abattoirs, who also has and lives with Asperger's), felt she could empathize more with cows than with people (see below).

B. TO COMPREHEND WHAT I SAW.

I also avoided looking at faces because of the meaningless of their component parts, [which] led to non-interpretable sensory-based behaviors and curiosity which were generally not welcomed.

If a face had no meaning, why stare? On the other hand, if she had little realization, as a child, of the way the face was connected to represent personhood, then staring would be natural.

I also did not like the shock of finding I had touched or stared at a part of someone's face and then realized that these parts belonged to the person. The jolt always disturbed me. I did not learn to stop touching or staring at people though I learned to stop touching hair, comparing noses and staring at blemishes. Another disturbance in looking at people was being echopraxic [mimicking their movements because they had taken over her actions], that I kept taking on their postures and facial expressions unintentionally, and this disturbed me and sometimes disturbed them.

It disturbed me because I just wanted to keep my own body connectedness intact and not have to have it trail off like that, like a wild horse. Sometimes others had more control over my body than I did and I did not like to experience that, when I realized I had slipped into involuntarily mimicking them.

We all have a body image, a conscious perceived self viewed as a whole, and a body schema, a nonconscious, preconscious system that coordinates sensory feedback and movement control to which we hardly attend. Ian, the subject who had lost all sensory feedback, had lost his schema and so had to attend, visually and mentally, to all movements. He used his body image as a replacement schema. Here, and in a later passage, she is suggesting that she did not have a body image, did not have a conscious and accessible sense of herself as a whole, as a person. She could walk and eat and so forth, without thought, according to stored repertoires, but was not aware of herself doing these things. She existed at the level of the body schema and occasionally had an image imposed on her by the presence of another, or from a mirror image.

Not comprehending facial expression is different to building up an ability to spot asymmetry and discrepancy. I could not read their faces, but I had a feel for the tone these faces had and if one part was out of sync from the rest it was like someone singing a flat note—it struck me. I did not read what someone felt, I read whether they were true to themselves (their connectedness), or whether they were trapped inside their bodies or could not dare expression. You have confused the two. Both are highly refined systems—one used by most people and one used by a handful of people who rely on sense and pattern and systems, rather than on interpretation.

Not being able to make consistent sense of facial expression also meant there was no consistent reward in what it was meant to express. Yes, this was worse with overload—it is a percentage thing. Overload could mean that thirty percent comprehension could slip to ten percent or nil. I also think that relying upon pattern and system sensing made reliance upon interpretation a late, acquired second language and so interpretation was generally a redundant system, because I already had one that I trusted far more in terms of my own social/emotional/perceptual/sensory reality. (I began to get some consistent interpretation around ten years old, by which time I was already a master of sensing).

D. ABOUT MOOD.

I could tell mood from a foot better than from a face. I could sense the slightest change in regular pace and intensity of movement of foot. I could sense any asymmetry in rhythm that indicated erraticness and unpredictability. I could sense the expressive from the reactive. Facial expression, by comparison, was so overlaid with stored expression, full of so many attempts to cover up or sway impression that the foot was much truer. I used sound in the same way, even breathing. Intonation aside, I could sense change in regular rhythm, pace, intensity and pitch. I think these things may be how animals make sense of people. Perhaps for them, as for me, this is a system that develops in the absence or delay of the development of interpretation.

Oliver Sacks found that Temple Grandin was more at home with and able to relate to animals than people:

We found a calm, quiet area of the farm, where cattle were browsing placidly. Temple knelt and held out some hay, and a cow came over to her and took the hay, nudging her hand with its soft muzzle. A soft, happy look came over Temple's face. "Now I'm at home," she said. "When I'm with cattle, it's not cognitive. I know what the cow's feeling . . . It's different with people . . ." (p. 256)[15]

Similarly perhaps, for Donna, people give too many confusing signals.

You ask about the back and forth flow. [I had asked about conversation, about the figure of eight relatedness between people talking to one another.] For me there is none. One thing that people find with me is that expression, rather than being constantly present, breaks through, as in bursts and this probably reflects system shifts and its effect on body connectedness and emotion. On a receptive level, my comprehension of the expression of others through their faces fluctuates in a similar way, though less so now with the lenses [Irlen lenses, which she has found enormously helpful in improving the processing of visual information]. Facial expression in my presence may be like bouncing a ball off a wall. The ball bounces back but nobody threw it.

Reciprocity in facial expression leads to a relationship, means we are "getting through." The returned smile shows a shared emotion. Here she describes pure imitation of expression with scarcely any connection to will, or want, or self. And without any self it does not reflect sharing, or a felt emotional response in its owner, if such a smile can be said to be owned. It is shown like a mirror's reflection, obeying the organic laws of physics she used to get by in our foreign world of emotion. Her smile did not reflect choice or engagement but quite the reverse.

> I do know that people who are glad to meet me become uncomfortable after a while because their outpouring receives no predictable feedback. On my part I have learned to stand there and put up with them until they get to their point, sometimes I cannot be bothered and I just walk off to something more interesting at the moment. It is a mechanical effort to continually attempt to remind myself that such actions may dent their feelings. Yet I just feel that they fill up time with auditory and visual waffle I cannot use in the immediate context in which it happens.

I had quoted the part of her book when she writes that someone kissed her face but she was not in it at the time. Where was she? I wrote about how sad I had felt to read of her problems with self in relation to others.

> Where did I reside, if not in my body? My body was often experienced as external and other. Some of this was due to system shift and shutdowns, so I lost body connectedness. I think that I could still be seen in my eyes sometimes. Sometimes my brain handled everything until my mind was redundant. Sometimes a reactive sort of database in me handled things and again my mind was redundant. Sometimes, I had emotions without mind. Sometimes, I had pure logic (mind) without emotion.

> Yes, the extinguishing of self merely because of the experience of others saddens me too. It is like in all my systems I have no modulation, no volume control, just an on/off switch.

> I am very grateful at least that, with my husband (Ian) I can experience him as an external part of me, so I relate to and experience him as self rather than other. This has its downfalls too—I sometimes, in an involuntary and compulsion driven state of self abuse, order him about as though he were "an out of control" body. I have smacked him as though his body was my own. Still, it works the same way for him too and he butts in on me, as though speaking with me as a part of his own self dialogue and he generally needs me with him in order to access his emotions and remain connected to his selfhood in the ocean of other. Often, mere presence can do this, but sometimes this works through eye contact—not that he sees what I feel as often I express nothing. It is for him like looking into a pool of water, which evokes connection with his selfhood. In that sense there is almost a benefit for him in my lack of physically connected selfhood and it works the same way for me.

The presence of another can be used to learn more of oneself. But for an autistic person this is only tolerable if that person is respectful of the other and allows them space.[16] Perhaps it is through relations with another, loved, one that we fully become aware of ourselves emotionally; perhaps that is an important part of what love is. Donna is suggesting that, even for an autistic person, eye contact is there and can have meaning, even when apparently expressing nothing. With her husband as an external part of her, the oneness of love is present. There *is* a difference between looking in the mirror and looking at him. On meeting Ian he suggested she tape over the mirrors that she had used for reassurance all her life, to try to get her further out into the world. He said, "It's a reflection . . . light bouncing from you onto the glass and being bounced back." For Donna, being "mono" made it "hard simultaneously to hold onto the logic when your perception told you it was another moving version of you." Her husband to be was becoming that moving and living version of her.

I had gone on to ask about her use of facial expression. Did it happen or did she control it?

> Yes, I have come to externally monitor my own facial expression. Through this I can often tell when a disconnected expression is on my face, but I can also tell when, much more occasionally, a connected emotion has made the physical connection to facial expression. I do feel that I have connected expression but it gets lost when experiencing other. I feel that in place of this, I learn to stick stored expressions on and over time, these became triggerable responses in response to patterns of behavior, though still disconnected to emotion—push button expression.

This has resonances with our own use of facial expressions. Sometimes we are happy or angry and show it, while at other times we feign expression—greeting someone we don't much care for warmly, for instance. These are our own disconnections which our multifaceted personalities can cope with.

In her childhood she had adopted certain characters, faces she showed the world. I asked about these.

E. MASKS.
> Mostly these are involuntarily triggered reactive stored repertoires. They can fill the void left by disconnection and even make the development of connection redundant. They do also protect from direct impact as well as suffocate the self from self expression and the building of relationships through familiarity. They are not about pretense, even though pretense is the closest word I probably had at the time. Pretense is intentional. Defensive, reactive, triggered, stored repertoires are not intentional. The only intention for me is in choosing not to fight them or to expose them for what they are.

I had asked about her ideas of the self and the face, and communication through facial expression and gaze.

Yes, gaze can capture a heart with trust, if that gaze is connected to the self within, and if there is a self honesty and self exposure in that gaze. Many people gaze with dead eyes, even if they might think they are true to themselves.

Self and face were not linked. Triggerable, reactive defence, like what comes out in disconnected facial expression is stored repertoire, the result of brain but not of mind. I distinguish between the brain (instinctual involuntary adaptations) and the mind (the self which has volition). The only point at which the mind comes into this is where it chooses to allow the adaptations of the brain to govern without a psychological fight.

I had asked if she felt any of the truth of Merleau-Ponty's saying about existing in another's facial expression.

I liked the Merleau-Ponty thing, if I exist in another's facial expression . . . Certainly, it was the reaction of others to my "characters' that encouraged reliance upon mechanical, disconnected expression in place of self expression, and helped develop a sort of defence of those characters as "selves."

Yet, for me, it was that rare experience of seeing in someone's eyes that they had seen me in there—beyond the suffocation of these distorting facades—that told me that I did exist. This was like oxygen to a flame about to go out and it fired the fight for expression of selfhood, for which I had almost exhausted all hope.

F. ABOUT "NOBODY HOME."
There is no thought of "oh, I will disconnect now," that is pretence. Shutdown gives no such choice. Shutdown is a product of the brain's adaptation to overload, it is not a product of mind. It is neurological, not psychological. This is where perhaps you can fathom out why I say I am not my autism, autism is not me. People with Asperger's syndrome sometimes defend that they are their autism. I know it shapes every fiber within me but it is no more me than if I were gripped by a virus. It is my developmental virus. It shaped my life but not my soul.

Being "at home" is not to do with feelings. It is to do with two things—one is body connectedness, but the other is connectedness of emotions and mind. If either of this is shut down or in a state of systems shift, the connection of selfhood and expression is either lost or generally unformed and socially incomprehensible.

Before my lenses [Irlen lenses filter out excessive visual information, reduce visual overload, and so make visual perception more cohesive, with spectacular results for both Donna and her husband], I did not recognize people by their faces any more than by their pace or pattern or form. I have been known to carry on a disrupted talk to someone because the person had the same hair or beard or glasses as someone else, and be shocked to find that the person does not know why I am talking to them. This is like recognizing the jigsaw by one of its pieces.

In dreams, too, faces did not figure much in recognition. Also in my paintings and drawings most are done with the subject facing away from the viewer. The only subjects that look at the viewer are cats. The rest have no living subjects in them. The expression of the cats in these pictures is through their direction of movement in relation to the viewer. One is specifically of a cat with "nobody home" in there.

A fragmented face expresses no self-honesty—it expresses nothing. Only in eyes can I see self-honesty—even then, I look from one eye to the other and generally cannot fathom out two at once, I'm mono-optic.

She went onto to explain why two way discourse was so difficult, and why, for her, cognitive theories about the problems of autism were inadequate.

G. BEING MONO.

Being mono [the experience of being able to keep hold of one system or one thing at once] makes it hard to hold simultaneous sense of self (internal feedback and reflection) and other (externally generated information requiring processing). Even in the absence of perceptual fragmentation, this form of mono can severely restrict processing of the response of others to oneself because, while a mono person is on an expressive track (involving accessing and monitoring the means of expression and the expression itself), they may not be able to simultaneously process incoming information for meaning and significance (such as the other person's responses to this expression).

You can see here how getting feedback regarding one's effect upon others can be severely restricted by this involuntary compensation of mono for managing information overload. Consider this, and [then] theory of mind . . . may have more to do with information processing, involuntary compensations, mono and perceptual problems than something so simplistic as being unable to imagine other minds.

It is self-other mono that is a real shit when it comes to identity and confidence in someone like me. So, I am not sorry that I know what these neurological bastards cost me. Here is perhaps a glimpse of that interplay between neurological problems and person-hood. Yes, it does shape personality to a degree and one's relationship to one's self and the world. It is so easy to confuse one's brain with one's mind and this has been one tangled ball of wool that I spent and still spend much of my life distinguishing between in order to remain as free and functioning and happy with life and my part in it as possible.

Autism for me is to do with having inefficient information processing, so that processing, accessing and monitoring involved in comprehension, response and self feedback is so delayed that everything comes in disconnected and in often meaningless bits and pieces. In this sense it is the perceptual and sensory problem to do with the brain and not the mind. I would say that I have neurological problems not mental problems. The brain is not the mind nor the ego. The brain does not decide it responds. The brain does not have preferences, simply some things that have functional priority. The brain does not give a damn about your (the person's, my) personal likes, dislikes or feelings. It would do what is instinctual to it, regardless of if it annoys or scares or compromises you (the person, me) socially or limits your (my) learning or cripples your (my) expression.

She returned to the somatic "body-centered" idea of self, to her body schema and image, and how—for her—she was most completely a person, most completely a mind, with and through art.

> I still do not feel right with the idea that I am my body, I have had the experience of this but it is not consistent. Mostly I think I exist in my sub-conscious or pre-conscious mind—not easily voluntarily accessible except through writing, music and painting. In daily life, my self is often inaccessible on a voluntary and conscious level, though it is certainly triggerable and able to be evoked. Much of my life is spent either writing, composing or in the company of someone with whom I feel safe to mirror or be triggered by. Mostly my direction is dictated by the things around me, rather than by conscious mind. I am stuck with this but if I go to winge [complain] all I have to do is to think about all the low functioning autistic people who do not have this adaptation. Then there is no winge.

I excused myself from the tea party and sat with her searing prose, moved by her revelations of what autism is for her and about her problems with theory of mind, with interpersonal relatedness, with the face, with other, and with the self. I had asked what I thought were some quite penetrating questions, not knowing if she and Paul (Ian in her books) would want or not want to reply. They had discussed these matters and more, and by their invitation to visit I hoped they had enough "want" to make it easier for them.

I drove to the sea in the west and stayed the night at a hotel close by. I booked in and went for a long run through the dark green hills, along roads and tracks bordered by small oaks forced to grow horizontal by the wind. It rained throughout the run, but it was warm rain with a soft breeze and I loved it. Through running I become as one, "mono" on my terms, with my own thoughts and my own feelings. Next morning there was time to run down to the Atlantic and gaze at the sea, lost in the waves rolling onto the rocks. I hoped I was ready to tune into whatever Donna and Paul were able to say.

She had explained in a letter that her interviews were all pre-scripted, in what she calls "read-speak." In some of her published interviews, in connection with her books, it was evident that the rules were more specific—no eye contact, no tape recorders (too noisy, I presumed: "NO, they cause too sharp awareness of 'other' that involuntarily clogs up the works in connection to expression with self intact"). They had given details of her life, the usual interview "blah, blah, blah" in Donna's idiosyncratic but accurate parlance. In contrast, I wanted to ask specific questions, knowing that to respond to conversation would be difficult. Maybe if I was less of a conversing presence, more a provoker of thoughts, it might be easier.[17] But still I would be trying to direct her and her husband's thoughts. Donna and Paul imposed no conditions on our meeting.

Just before the visit Paul rang to give some last arrangements. How would they recognize me? What would I be wearing? My concerns must have been evident, for he ended, "Don't be nervous, because that makes us nervous too." At the time arranged they drove to meet me. I was the only person waiting. I came out to greet them and then followed them back to their house in my car. Paul had asked over the phone who I looked like. I had said, modestly, Clint Eastwood. When I got to their house Donna told me she thought I reminded her of the person in Munch's *The Scream*.

I had asked if I might see her paintings, and bring some favorite works of my own, for I wondered if we might converse through art. Over the phone she had said that she was an expressive artist, not a receptive one, but had agreed to try it. She offered me a chance to look at their pictures: Paul's were strong and precise drawings of buildings and engineering. Donna's, by contrast, were impressionistic, free, and almost abstract. The portraits were there, with the subjects facing away from the viewer, into the wall. I thought of Munch's gentle aquatint, *The Lonely One* (1896), also with the subject facing away. One an artistic device to express alienation perhaps, the other a necessity. Donna showed me another painting of hers. "Can you see what it is?" I could see swirls but could not make out what they represented. A wheat field perhaps? "Hens." Then I could see the head and bodies of chickens, dark and difficult to extract from the morass of background. She was teaching me something about visual overload. She showed me Klimt's *Birkenwald, 1903,* a depiction of beech woods so clear it is almost unnerving for me.

"Artists? I don't like any nor love any. I saw Klimt's painting. That was our visual processing exactly without the Irlen lenses. That excited us both but not out of like, it was out of knowing there was something others could observe that would show them what it was like. Unlike Van Gogh or Monet, his painting showed not just the visual fragmentation but the chaos. Most paintings by other people impose a sense of 'other' on the viewer. They have a sense of intent or direction that pokes at you like unwelcome fingers and robs you of your right to find freely what you would in them. The paintings seem to dictate how you look at them and in this way they rob you of self in their imposition of other and, in my case, leave no self left with which to weigh up the experience of such paintings."

I had wondered if a static face was easier than a moving one, since less information was being expressed.

"In terms of visual processing a static face is easier. In terms of self-other mono, generally not. Both the static face and the moving face generally impose a sense of other at the expense of connection to sense of self. The static one is socially easier to handle, though, because it won't blah at you or grab you and try to force eye contact. The static face of a picture is controllable and able to be abandoned without consequence. That's why I choose to spend time with statues. I have seen paintings of distorted faces. They sometimes express a feeling of brutality—like as if someone took the privilege of order and intentionally tore it to shreds to indulge in constructed chaos. That goes in the opposite direction to the motivation my autism drives me to."

I had come with a book of Velasquez and one of Bacon. The Bacon I kept in my bag.[18] I showed her the massive portraits of Velasquez. She looked at Pope Innocent X and Sebastian de Gorra, a dwarf. Both must be well off, she thought, by looking at their clothes. She commented on the second being a dwarf and I told her of how they were kept by the royal court. She looked at the portraits but said little more. I explained the captured power and cruelty of the Pope, the terror he could generate in others, and the dignity and self-knowledge that Velasquez had captured in the dwarf. I turned to his portrait of Calabazas, another court jester. She immediately saw that he was blind (so she *had* looked at the eyes), but added no more. Portraits were evidently not a way of connecting. Then I sat down with her comments on my earlier manuscript. Paul offered me a drink and as I drank I read, while Donna and he discussed other matters with themselves and with a house guest. I was absorbed in her comments and happy to be there without imposing.

I had asked how she had been so precise in her description of her self from her photos in *Nobody Nowhere*. She had explained that,

I can see connection or disconnection to self in a collection of photos of others. I can also see the system used to manage overload through viewing collections of photos of a particular person.

I can see a smile or a crumpled up face. I can see tears. I can see nobody home.

I generally can't see or have little idea why people have particular expressions on their faces.

Was I remembering what I was like or reading facial expression? Remembering and then seeing it was captured by the camera which confirmed the validity of memory—especially given that I'd been told I was mad—so I didn't trust memory unless it was confirmed.

I was intrigued about the creative process in her writing. Was it semiconscious or preconscious? Did she gain any satisfaction from it? I had written of my astonishment that a writing savant can be so insightful, yet has so little organized self. Writing, I had asked, is it a dialogue with herself, or does it just come out from nowhere, or is it a dialogue with people you cannot stand to converse with in other ways? She replied that it was at one level monologue, at another a dialogue with herself which evades consciousness. It does come from her, but could be used more impersonally, a preconscious freed monologue that her conscious mind is excluded from until the reading of what comes out; thought in print form, untranslated.

This led to my next question, for it seemed that it was only in art that she was fully able to express herself or connect, or truly "be." I asked if it was a semiaware skill. Was she was able to gain any satisfaction from it?

It is the process of musical composition, writing, or art that is automatic so it has no conscious connection nor experience. The product of that process—the actual words being read back, the music being heard back, the picture as each fragment emerges in the sculpturing of a painting—these I have conscious monitoring and experience of but being excluded from the process, it is like being given "gifts" by another within me so the word "satisfaction" is wrong. "Satisfaction" is a word to do with whether one is pleased with what the process produced. To feel this, one must have an "expectation" of what one wishes to come out. There must be "trying" or "intention." Consciously I have none of these so "satisfaction" is entirely irrelevant and unfitting as if someone showed me by surprise someone else's beautiful and impacting painting and said, "are you, Donna, satisfied with it?" My answer would be, "I find it sensorily pleasing" or "it touches me" or "I feel belonging with this painting" but it would be disconnected and false to say, "I am satisfied with this" for the "I" in this sentence (me) had no conscious experience of its creation nor the intent from which it sprung.

After I had finished reading, Donna and Paul came in and we discussed matters from the writing, and matters like the absence of theory of mind in some autistic persons. (She thought the theories correct but irrelevant—when you grow up without something, then you get by with other methods and live under different rules. It is those different rules that should be studied and understood in order to help autistic people, rather than concentrating on what they do not have.) We talked of how best to allow autistic people to live: in a world apart from "typicals," or in a more tolerant and wider yet equal society? By speaking quietly and looking mainly at the table or wall in front of me while Donna stood above me—or walked animatedly, urgently around—we conversed. Paul, busy next door, would come in occasionally to make a point. Donna would often use a set of figures of cows as people, to elaborate, moving them in front of me across the table.

In both my letters and now I gently raised questions of them together. Was there any sense that some part of what attracted and led to love was seen through the face, in the sense that the face represented the person?

"Not a whole face because I could not perceive one but there was 'Paul's nose,' 'Paul's eyebrow,' 'Paul's eye,' and for him there was 'Donna's nose,' and so forth. We knew each other as collections of these component parts. We were married after having seen each other only once as whole bodies and whole faces, through Irlen lenses, but before we actually got them sent to us, so we actually married as we had lived— with no cohesive impression of each other—just a cohesive sense of each other and a fragmented impression. What led to love was that cohesive sense that came from its fragments and from pattern. Yes, even if I could take only one eye at a time, I was struck, as with my younger brother, by his trappedness and pattern of connection and disconnection but not feeling for him, but feeling for the me in his form (that is to do with my concept of 'me' being a fragmented one that this is possible for me, but maybe not so possible for others who conceive of themselves daily and moment by moment as a whole self)."

She talked of how being able to be with someone, loving him, depended on that person not taking too much from her, allowing her "self" to exist, by not invading or taking from her the fragile "me." Love then came from knowledge of there being two such people, respecting each other mutually, independently. I was reminded of Kahlil Gibran's famous simile of love being like two strings of a violin, separate yet united in their playing of music. I thought of how much we had to learn from them both.

Time was getting on. I knew that to talk with a stranger was difficult for them both. She had suggested two hours of "blah, blah, blah" was all she could take, and the time was over. Paul had almost finished preparing lunch, and they wondered aloud what to do with "him." I said that I had to leave, for I was driving that day to the opposite end of England with my family to see my sister and brother-in-law. Donna gave a yelp of delight at my going, then corrected herself, saying it was nothing personal.

As I went out into their courtyard, Donna skipped and danced her way around it, beautiful as a child or young foal is beautiful, wrapped up in her delight in movement. I felt she was connected, hoped she was. She came back, and looking at the ground in front of me, said that she realized how difficult it was to understand their world but that she thought I would do it well. I thanked her for the morning and for her time in corresponding, and most of all for her compliment, which I would not forget. Then she was off.

As I got into the car Paul came up. "You know, Donna and I never look at each other's faces. We have our own private communication and language." I thanked him for all his help and drove off to our busy family world and its glorious social soup. Private, I thought, Donna and Paul's shared world should remain private.

I had been drawn to autism by the most circuitous of routes. Stuck with ecological theories of facial action based on primate work, I wanted to construct ideas about the face as more than a displayer of social signals. I had gone to see primates for myself looking for a way out of this, for a way of restoring the face as the site of expression of mood and feelings. With facial expression came ways into other minds and a social existence. Theory of mind allowed this, but such a *theory*, an explanation rooted in the cognitive thinking world—though ingenious and useful—did not seem to encompass all that the face did, nor explain all that the evolution of faces allowed. The face, our human face, seemed a way of reaching people, of relating to them, of feeling toward which was quite unlike that seen in most other animals.

In autistic persons this relating and empathy toward was absent, strikingly, and their reflections on such a life, and on a life without the empathetic face, seemed a useful and important reflection allowing us to understand, at one remove, something of what the face represents.

Donna clearly describes the way in which facial conversations involve and depend on a relation and engagement between two or more people. For most of us this is welcoming and warming, but for shy people this can be disturbing and for autistic persons it is almost overwhelmingly threatening to their fragile selfhood. They actively avoided faces because of their vulnerability to be taken over by others in the figure of eight that is facial conversation. This contrasted with talking, which was evidently easier and allowed conversation with a necessary independence for self-preservation. Looking at others led to an emotional engagement and to an engulfment, "an extinguishing," of self and to the experience of scarcely controllable internal emotions, poorly expressed by body language, facial expression, and language, and so poorly controlled. For with little ability to express inner feeling states, those emotions themselves are distorted and threatening. In describing a disconnectedness from her body, a lack of embodiment, in part due to an absence of facial expressiveness, there was no channel for the expression and the true experience, and hence control, of emotion.

Yet there were other reasons for avoidance. Faces, for instance, gave too many signals. Faces make many subtle movements simultaneously, too many for autistic persons to process. A single expression, like a simple musical theme, might be learned and understood by rote, but the complex, almost symphonic use of the face we all engage in was just too difficult. These many and subtle movements may have explained why Donna found deception in the facial expressions of others, in those faces she described as being not true to their self.

Donna's firsthand account obviously has its limitations. For anyone to disentangle the problems associated with sensory overload and the effects this has on emotional development and sense of self and of others, to overcome the "neurological bastards," must be extraordinarily difficult. But, given these problems, her own account of her experience and her responses to my questions did have an internal consistency. Her world, though so different from our own, was intelligible to me. By focusing on her problems with facial expressions I gained understandings of autism unavailable in complementary, more objective, accounts. Just as important, with these insights came reflections on the use of the face in us "typicals," which would otherwise not have been obtained.

But autism, of course, is a widespread developmental disorder, not just a face thing. Do the many other problems they have preclude too many conclusions about relatedness and social development based on facial action? Perhaps. But what if there were people with facial problems alone, and what if they experienced some similar difficulties in relatedness? Autism is a condition with problems in social interaction which are reflected in problems with the face. What if we could turn this upside down? How might facial problems affect social development and selfhood?

The Spectator

Those with autism had not been supposed to attend to the face: corresponding with Donna Williams had allowed me to understand why this was and, in turn, had allowed some insight into both autism and the face. To live with autism is not to be devoid of emotion either, rather to be full of emotions but with little ability to understand or express them.

So I went next to talk with a group of people whose condition is almost exclusively facial. But first it was necessary to explore some of the past work on the way in which an infant's development might be linked to her face. It soon became apparent that one way we first go out into the world as babies, learn about it, and learn to influence others is through the face.

Imitation, Self, and Others

Though hand movements in imitation occur relatively early in a child's life, facial imitation was thought, until recently, to occur only after around eight to twelve months.[1] For infants to make facial movements they have to connect the self and the other in a unique way. They have to perform an act, the pulled face, seen in another with an act—their own pulled face—which they cannot see, and this was thought beyond them in their early months.

In 1977 Meltzoff and Moore, however, showed that facial imitation can take place in the first days of life.[2] They went on to find infants in whom simple imitation of tongue protrusion and mouth opening occurred after forty-two minutes. Within days babies can distinguish their mother's face from a stranger's.[3] The child, seeing the adult's face, must gain feedback from her own facial muscles and skin of her own facial movement in response to another's visual act. This was the aspect which previous investigators had neglected, for as adults can feel internally facial position and movement (a process called proprioception), using information from the skin and muscles of the face, so can infants. Not only that, babies can make faces, and learn faces, at extraordinarily early ages. The conclusion had to be that this was happening in a preprogrammed innate system.[4,5]

Why should this imitative skill be present so early? Are they just reflexes, to kid the adult that his child is cute and smart and so encourage care, but meaningless for the baby herself? Perhaps not, for a baby will give the face posed for one adult to the next one she sees; the baby *remembers* facial expressions. Babies, as every parent knows, struggle to produce these expressions and learn, through getting them wrong, how to make the best faces. They lie there practicing, they try them out on their carers; their faces are the first part of the body that they take an interest in controlling, not just to suck, but to express. Meltzoff and Moore suggested that infants learn something of people through and by imitation, enacting their actions, and that this early imitation represents not motor reflexes but early social interaction and cognition. The beginnings of individuality and personality may arise from these early facial learnings.

Facial expressions and learning, however, may also have deeper effects than this. Through imitation a face can be assimilated from visual experience, through proprioception, into felt experience: something can be taken from being "out there" in another, to being in me.[6] Certain faces can then be given a context; faces look like what the infants feel themselves to be. For facial movements are not like movements of an arm or a leg; they straddle the uncertain boundaries of movement, behavior and internal states or moods. Through the face a child may map externally perceived behavior onto a set of internal bodily impressions. If mental states are located in the mind, and physical ones in and on the body, then facial movements may lie between the two, movements with a relation to internal states. Next comes initiation; babies soon learn not just to respond but to influence and manipulate others. Within a few months they can initiate and discontinue shared visual attention.[7]

If we are born alone it is through the face that we first experience things out there that are like us, that respond to us, and which, by making faces, we can influence. It is through movement of the face that we first learn about others and about ourselves. Babies produce faces they see others perform and may use them as identifiers of who they are and use reenactments to confirm this. They are working out problems and attending to some faces and neglecting others. From these early choices they are imposing meaning on experience. All this appears to be going on while the infant may be unable to control her head, or sit, or do much more than wave the arms and legs around in a swimming or flying motion. Yet they stare at their carers, gurgle, and smile or frown, cry and grimace. The control of the face far exceeds control of other parts. For a baby—prelingual and with few useful movements and little body language—the face and eyes are the site, almost the only site, of communication not just of bodily needs but for the beginnings of individualization and character formation.

It is through the sharing of facial expressions that mother and child become as one. It is crucial, in a more Darwinian biological context, for the infant to bond her mother to ensure her own survival. The sharing of life and of experience, which is the joy of parenthood, begins in the face. Within an individual's lifetime the face is perhaps most important in the first weeks and months of life.

Child's Play

This reliance on the face is given in the way in which mothers and fathers and siblings, and anyone else, will greet a baby with an exaggerated slow and obvious smile, inviting the baby to share his or her joy and reflect it. In the first few weeks and months facial expressions given by mothers to their babies are exaggerated in both space and time. A mother will give a huge mock surprised look, eyes wide open, mouth agape, and eyebrows up, when the baby turns to her. She holds this expression for longer than in adult conversations, as though in slow motion. Mothers offer fewer expressions but exaggerate them. They use a big frown, a concern/sympathy pantomime, a rather neutral face, and of course—and most of all—a big smile. Stern[8,9] suggests that these allow the mother and baby to initiate, maintain, modulate, and to terminate social interactions. Surprise initiates, the smile maintains, and the frown terminates, while the neutral face, especially with gaze aversion, signals lack of intent to engage.

The rules for mutual gaze appear to be different in mothers and babies compared with adults. Grown-ups rarely gaze into each others' eyes without speech for more than a few seconds, unless they are about to fight or make love. In contrast, mother and child remain engaged for thirty seconds or more, and during play a mother may gaze at her baby for seventy percent of the time. Taking turns during speech is also very different. In adults we look at the speaker most of the time, while during speech we look away. During play a mother will gaze and speak simultaneously. During feeding she will look but not speak, so as not to disrupt the feeding. In peekaboo and many other games a major element in play is face presentation and expression.

For the first few weeks of life a baby will spend much of her waking life feeding and being cleaned, and during these activities the child will be inches from her mother's eyes. The mother's face is the first place the baby's gaze is directed toward, the first place a child learns about human relatedness.[10]

At about six weeks of age the baby can fix the mother's eyes and hold her gaze. The mother becomes aware that her baby is really looking at her. This alters as the child grows and begins to become independent. The relationship begins to involve two people rather than one giving all to the other. By three months the infant's visual system has matured to be able to see farther away and the infant can now track across a room, extending the distance over which gaze can be used to regulate engagement. The baby can also begin to choose when and whom to look at. Slowly, by the end of the first six months, the baby is beginning to look for objects to play with. The preeminence of the face may have been lost until the child falls in love again, this time as an adult, but its importance in many aspects of communication remains.

At about eight months of age infants become distressed when separated from their mother. After this, however, there is a slackening of this bond which allows development with other persons, relatives, and friends. Children need to learn about others, develop social skills, relate to their peers, get on at school. While linguistic and cognitive skills become of more importance, the affective emotional part of ourselves remains paramount.

In the Playground

There has been much work on what determines how popular a child is with his or her peers. Antony Manstead and Roselyne Edwards[11] reviewed evidence on the way in which children learn to recognize facial expression in others from still photographs, paralleling their own development of increasingly subtle facial expressiveness. Three- to-five-year-olds could only reliably recognize happiness; anger was recognized at age seven, fear by ten, and surprise by eleven. Errors in matching of faces to emotions suggested that younger children had broader conceptions of emotion categories, so that in three-year-olds "mad" was most often confused with "scared" or "disgusted." Though there are obvious linguistic as well as emotional problems to be overcome in such experiments, the findings do suggest an increasing accuracy in emotion matching in children as they grow up.[12]

One of the more important findings from this work is that there are large variations in these tasks between children of the same age. Do these variations have any effect on peer popularity? The ability to recognize facial expression accurately in others turns out to be a predictor of emotional competence, defined in terms of the ability to discern one's own and others' feelings, and to respond sympathetically to others. Not surprisingly this, in turn, was correlated with peer group popularity. In contrast, poor recognition was associated with higher levels of delinquency and school dropout. Now, of course, it is not known if these relationships are causal, so Manstead and Edwards set up a long-term study which looked at emotion recognition, by facial expression and peer group popularity, in a group of 170 children, aged five to seven years. The emotions were given in photographs of faces and peer group popularity was determined by asking children whom they liked to play with, or whom they would ask to their birthday party. They concluded that a child's popularity at five helped to account for her emotion recognition ability at seven, even when differences in emotion recognition at five are taken out: popularity helps shape emotion recognition. But how well a child recognizes facial expressions at five also predicts how popular a child will be at seven, when differences in popularity at five are discounted, suggesting that emotion recognition plays a part in peer group popularity. It works both ways, in the playground, at seven years of age. If you are at the top of your peer group and everyone likes you, you learn to recognize faces well and respond accordingly. Knowing your facial expressions well (and hence other's moods) helps you get on with people. While no one would suggest that facial expression recognition is the key to world success or domination, it has been shown to play a part in early development and may also be part of later development of friendships and other relationships.

The Reflection of Ourselves

We have seen that we gain feedback about ourselves from the responses of others as we enter into relationships. Yet we also receive internal feedback from muscle and skin movement in the face. Might this neural feedback activity contribute to our own mood and emotion?[13] And if our emotions are to any extent determined by the expression of them, can we alter the former by controlling the latter? This almost Stanislavskian technique, in which the actor imagines himself or herself either to be the person being portrayed, or experiencing the same situation as that person, was anticipated by the eighteenth-century German playwright Gotthold Lessing,[14] and was known to Darwin, who wrote in his book on expression,

The free expression, by outward signs, of an emotion intensifies it. On the other hand repression, as far as this is possible, of all outward signs softens our emotions. He who gives way to violent gestures will increase his rage: he who does not control the signs of fear will experience fear in a greater degree and he who remains passive when overwhelmed with grief loses his best chance of recovering elasticity of mind.[15]

This passage suggests both that expression intensifies emotion and that control of some emotions, during the grief process, can be a bad thing, something now recognized far better than in Victorian days.

William James went further. For him facial expressions helped define emotion; the emotion was its physical expression.[16] If a passion was not expressed, then it would not occur, or if once expressed was stopped, then it would die. More recently, Fridlund reviewed the evidence for this "facial feedback hypothesis" and found none of it convincing.[17] He used examples which, however, were necessarily limited: Bell's palsy, in which one side of the face is paralyzed; and drug-induced temporary muscular paralysis. Neither provided evidence for changed mood and emotion following reduced facial movements, but both were unusual situations and unlikely to reflect natural functioning.

Adelmann and Zajonc[18] were much more convinced, and cited experiments in which subjects posed emotion while looking at a scene or film and rating it as sad or happy. Those posing a smile rated the film funnier than those posing a grimace. In one ingenious paper the subjects viewed a cartoon with a pen in their mouth, either between the lips (thus preventing smiling) or between the teeth (thus enabling, even facilitating, smiling). The latter group found the film funnier. All such studies, however, have many drawbacks, not least that a posed smile is hardly natural.

Perhaps if one had never known facial feedback, one's experience would have been different, though what might then be due to the experience of others and to reduced facial feedback might be difficult to disentangle. I went to speak with a rare group of people who have never known feedback from movement of their faces and have never experienced what it is to smile or to frown. John Hull had talked of those who cannot move their faces as having a curious kind of priestly witness, of suggesting that all things are not necessary for human life. I went to see one such priest.

James

"I'll tell you about my family. I was born in 1939, the third of six brothers and sisters. I was tongue-tied and the family doctor, who was a surgeon, did a series of operations releasing it. At the same time they had to find a way of feeding me. Eventually they used the inside of a fountain pen and dripped it into my mouth. I am told that each feed took two hours, and then I was sick and they did it again. My parents had a nurse who was living in at each of these confinements and she stayed longer, far longer than the usual month to help. In the family circle I was regarded as just another member of the family. I don't think I had any awareness of being different at all until I moved out of the family circle when I was eight and went to the village school. I was very late because of the things which were happening to me.

"The school, in the 1940s, in Staffordshire, in a rural area, was a true village school. It had the children of farmers, schoolmasters, all mixed in together. It wasn't a cruel environment but it was tough. I did begin to realize then that I was not quite like other children. Occasionally, at home, I used to salivate when I talked and sometimes I was accused of spitting when there was no intention to do so. That cropped up again at school. They used to say that I had spat in the cocoa or that I was spitting at some other boy and I'd get into trouble. I don't think it had occurred to me inside the family environment that there was anything particularly unusual about me. What made me realize that I was different was the questioning about my funny face, which I don't remember as being insistent, but it did crop up from time to time.

"At the age of eleven, when I went to the grammar school, I used to be asked why do I cry when I eat because the tear ducts which behaved themselves at other times lacrimated with food. They still do and I have to wipe my face. My father was a schoolmaster at the grammar school and my older brother was at the top end of the school. In those early years I was teased, partly because my father was on the staff and my older brother was a senior pupil; people wanted to get at me because of that, not simply because of the face. It may not have had anything to do with myself and I think I misunderstood that. I was an object of curiosity and interest, not simply because of what I was but because of who I was. I did, however, begin to become aware of difficulties in communicating with people. For instance, in those early years at grammar school some people didn't understand me. If I put my hand up in class because I knew the answer, the teacher wouldn't ask me. Some of the masters were afraid they wouldn't understand what I said. I felt neglected.

"I had some speech therapy for two or three years. The speech therapist helped me considerably in slowing down and separating the words. She taught me to put the final consonant onto the end of a word to help people understand what I was saying. By the time I got near the top end of the school some of the masters had become used to me. By the end of my time at grammar school, masters would say that while it wasn't exactly a pleasure to talk to you at least we could understand what you're saying. It was a single-sex school and we lived about seven miles outside town. Whatever disadvantages or difficulties I had because of my face, I also had the difficulty in socializing because my friends lived in town and there was only one bus home and I had to be on it. It was only when I was in the sixth form that I started going to one or two out-of-hours gatherings of different kinds and I started to get about. I was afraid and in awe of girls for a long time.

"I was fairly placid as a child but I sometimes remember my face working for me rather than against me. If I did something wrong I'd say 'It wasn't me mummy, it was him,' my brother thirteen months younger, and I would be believed. I soon learned that my facial problem could allow me deception. I've never played poker. As a child I did a lot of reading, which suggests a certain solitary quality. In my teens I read a lot of Hardy, which was perhaps not the ideal thing at that stage either for me or for others around me. I would be by myself in the book burying my face in it.

"I had always had it in mind to offer myself for ordination and when I was around eighteen I had an interview and was offered a place at Cambridge as long as I was accepted by the Church as a candidate for ordination. So I went to a Church of England Selection Conference which recommended in turn that I should be taken on for training. I had the medical in Chester which I failed on the grounds of speech. The standing and walking were also thought to be too much of an obstacle. It was a great shock to have passed the theological interview and yet have the doctor turn me down. I remember that. But there was a second opinion built into the process and I went to see a Harley Street man at the Church's expense. He said, 'Well, Mr. Brown, I can understand you, and you walked across my extensive consulting room well enough,' so he reversed the decision.

"I talked to my sister, who is five years older than me, about the time I was rejected, and she said that when the first doctor rejected me there was extreme consternation both at home and in the village—and an anger, which I had forgotten. I have a great capacity for forgetting things. It isn't just ordinary forgetfulness. I was eighteen and I don't think I would have forgotten it just out of simple forgetfulness.

"Meeting people in an interview situation I thought of as a hurdle that had to be got over, or an ordeal that had to be endured. Such matters were not so difficult as those areas which are voluntary. I was always better at things which had to be done rather than things that might be done."

James had reached the age of eighteen in his story without really focusing on his facial problem, a rare condition called Möbius syndrome, named after Paul Möbius (1853–1907), a German neurologist. Diane Williams, an American nurse who has the syndrome, wrote of her problems in a paper published in 1986.[19] "I am unable to raise my eyebrows, close my eyes tightly, move my eyes to the side, smile or move my lips . . . my face has a mask-like appearance." This description befits James too, as does Möbius' original case. James cannot move his facial muscles, and has rather drooping and wide eyes, with a narrow open mouth. He has no sideways movement of the eyes, so that in order to gaze at something, or someone, he has to move the whole head. I reminded James that he had hardly mentioned his face.

"I have a notion which has stayed with me over much of my life— that it is possible to live in your head, entirely in my head. Whether that came out of my facial problem I don't know. I was very introspective. I divided people into two categories: those who didn't want to have anything to do with me for various reasons and those who did. I think I had a low idea of self-worth. Thinking about it and reflecting upon it, I think in a sense a Christian shouldn't think too highly of himself in any case, though I realize you do not have to belittle yourself either."

"But loving one's neighbor as oneself requires, *presupposes* that you love oneself."

"Yes, I've struggled with that. I haven't related these things to my face particularly and that's why I haven't been speaking about it. I just haven't focused anything on the face. I had feelings of low self-esteem and loneliness and isolation in company, where I wasn't with anyone particularly, and I had the feeling, say, at a long table with a meal going on around me that the conversation divided around me and I was left on my own to eat my food and I was happy to do that, but not really happy—these feelings I have lived with, in my head. I always found it difficult to break in."

"An open, smiling face, for instance, is an invitation to come to a person."

"It is only very recently that the whole area of nonverbal communication has even come to my attention. I know now that since I put out a reduced range of signals I receive back a similarly reduced range. Impoverishment: there is a degree of uncertainty. Is he going to know me today, is he going to speak to me today, as I approach someone in the street? As I go about in the High Street I see people coming toward me and I can tell if they're going to get ready to speak to me if I speak to them, but it has taken me a long time to latch onto that fact."

"By deciding to live in your head, and ignoring the face problem, you turned away from others and did not present any part of you to the world. Is that fair?"

"Yes. Whether or not that was because of the shock which I experienced when I moved out of the family circle, where I was accepted and treated normally, or not, I don't know. It was a great shock, though I can only view it in those terms now. Whether that decision of mine to ignore things was a way of dealing with the situation I don't know."

"Was your facial problem ever mentioned at interview?"

"No. Very rarely has anyone ever mentioned my lack of expression or my facial appearance to me. I think I was lonely at Cambridge. Again I don't relate it to my face, although it may be pertinent. I lived in digs in my first year, I made one or two friends among the theological students. I didn't join a lot of societies. The first year I was quite lonely. The second and third years I was resident in college and that was far better—in the center of things."

I thought how difficult it must have been to project any self-esteem in college with such a problem as Möbius. Yet James seemed not to relate these difficulties to his face at all. I asked to what extent he thought his lack of facial expression affected this.

"I don't really think in those terms even now. You just accept that that's the way you are without asking why.

"I didn't like the cross-country traveling to get to and from Cambridge. So after three years of it I wanted to be closer to home and I went to theological college in Lichfield. After a year or so the bishop brought me in. He was a tremendous man, six feet five inches, rowed for Cambridge in the thirties. He said, 'Now look, Brown, I want everything to be done that can be done so that when I present you to a parish

I can say that everything has been done. Then I can say, "Love him and get on with it.'"

"So I went to the National Hospital in London and I was investigated and had some electrodes attached to me. The consultant explained the connection between the condition of the feet and the face. He explained to me that the muscles were in working order but the nerves were not. He said there was some movement in the eyes, up and down, but less from side to side. The only thing he said that could be done then was to use a muscle graft to attach to the corners of the mouth to create some sort of smile, but at that stage he said they couldn't guarantee that it would be equal. He said that he didn't think that it was a good idea. I was happy not to have an operation and didn't go for it. I think I made the right decision.

"The doctor showed me off to his group of students saying, I remember, 'It's worth having a look at this person because you may never meet such a person in all your years of practice.' This did me good because I could think, 'Oh, it's rare,' slightly humorously. You see, that's an area of difficulty. People tend to take everything I say seriously, for the reason that I can't smile. I can't always communicate a joke—it's all to do with facial expression and I've got into trouble because of that. I say things with a straight face. Once a young woman asked me what I'd do as a curate if a young baby cries at a baptism and I said, 'Oh, I'd hit its head on the side of the font,' and she went to the vicar with great anger and upset because she didn't realize that I was in fact joking."

It is difficult to imagine not being able to express frivolity and worse, perhaps, not being expected to even feel frivolous.

"I did want to be ordained at the time but a kind of expectation builds up in a long period of training and once you set out along that road it takes a lot of courage to get off it again. If you fail, then that does it for you, but if you keep going and you pass one milestone after another—it's like being engaged: there's tremendous expectation that it will arrive at marriage. I think I remember an element of that through university and theological college. Ordination was not perhaps the joy it might have been because I was simply doing something which had come to be expected.

"After ordination I went to a parish in the Black Country near Wolverhampton. A big town parish and the bishop said, 'I want you to go to this parish, go and see the vicar.' He said nothing else and I went to see the vicar and he had two boys with hare lips and cleft palates, two out of three. I came back and said to the bishop that I would be happy to go to that parish, partly because I was of that mind, that if the bishop said, 'Go there,' then I would go there. He said, 'I didn't tell you anything before you went, but you will have gathered that the vicar has two sons with harelips and cleft palates so he is familiar with some of the problems that you have, so he may be helpful.' I was very appreciative of that. I thought, here is a bishop who had a reputation for caring greatly about his clergy who has worked things out in some detail.

"I liked this vicar and his wife, and for around eighteen months I was quite happy there. I don't think too much was asked of me or demanded of me. I do remember that it was an effort to walk down the road with not only the face but the dog collar and cassock; the face and the uniform, to walk down the road, to make visits, to talk to people. Unfortunately this vicar accepted the offer of a move, which he was quite entitled to do, so after eighteen months a new vicar came to the parish whom I felt I didn't get on with so well. We had a professional relationship, whereas the previous vicar was a friend and had befriended me."

"Were you available to befriend people? You said it in a passive voice, as though others befriended you. You weren't able to go out to them?"

"It's much more difficult to go out to them. Yes. And that's occurred over and over again. Some days I could go out and see four or five people, some days I'd sit at home, not able to do it. I interpreted that as being not very good at the job. I was judgmental on myself about this."

"Yet you chose a job that made you go out into the world. What aspects of the job of becoming a vicar appealed to you?"

"I think the aspect of leading worship. Much of course is invisible—until you're ordained you don't really know what it involves. As a child you saw the local vicar at church, not in the community. I was attracted to that. That's odd. Why did it attract me if I had difficulty in speech and communication? Possibly a captive audience. It may be that I was looking for a fixed social role to play in front of others. I did enjoy talking with and listening to a group of older people, say in their homes, and taking the odd funeral and that's still true today. I feel that worked. I feel that today in a way that some of the other things didn't work. Chairing meetings for instance, I was much less happy to do. I'm not someone who can get their way.

"It was a conscious effort to go out and meet new people, say a new family moving into the parish. I had a social role which to some extent I hid behind. Well, I thought I did, but it is in that area that I became uncertain. I lost that sense of myself. Perhaps I lost it so long ago but I became aware of the fact that I didn't have that sense of myself.

"I met Anne in my first parish. She was one of the congregation and I came to know her because I was lodging with someone who was a friend and a distant relation. She used to call on my landlady and was thrust at me. I found the first few days after we met very difficult, but I had a very practical reason for persisting: the landlady had left for six weeks and I found it difficult to cope. Of course I was taken with her as well and have always been very glad that we both persisted. Once we began to relax together, then we both were fairly equally committed and there was a reciprocity which was entirely different. I think initially, was I thinking I was in love with her or feeling it? I was probably thinking it initially. It was some time later when I realized that I really felt in love."

"When did you realize that what was wrong with you had a name? When did you realize that there were others?"

"Extraordinarily, only recently when my mother-in-law saw an article in *Weekly News* by Linda Anderson about her son. She sent me the cutting. When I read his story, about a little boy who can't smile, I recognized myself. That was the first time that I had realized that there were others, really like me.

"At Cambridge and later I think I survived by being withdrawn or introspective. I made a virtue of keeping myself to myself. I think I rather liked being not like the others. You can become very perverse. For far too long that's what I did. I liked being not like the others. I gained some solace from it."

"Were you deceiving yourself?"

"Yes, I think so. I got into various difficulties later on because it wasn't a way of coping over a lifetime. It worked for quite a long time. Maybe it worked until my mother died in 1980, when I was in my forties. When she died I think I began a very slow process of reflecting on the relationship and my life and what I really wanted to do and I think I discovered things that led to my retirement. I remember that I realized that I didn't really want to do what I was doing. I had a depressive illness after my mother died. I went to see a psychiatrist and had a lot of help. The psychiatrist was also a priest so I found the right man.

"More recently, for the first time, I've been talking to someone, a spiritual director, and he asked me about anger and my condition, and that had never really occurred to me. Are you angry with God? Can you ever forgive Him? And I think, yes, I have been angry. Maybe in other things that I've tried and failed my anger has found expression, but I haven't related it to the face."

"To be angry and yet not express anger—"

"Part of the problem is that you're not supposed to. If you're angry you're told to stop it; but it is a powerful emotion and I realize that now, and that it can do a lot of damage. I think it did do a lot of damage in the relationship between my wife and I, and in my attitude to work and parishioners. I came to think that I had to choose between the role of being a vicar and myself. I went to a counselor and in conversation with him I realized that I had to make a choice, and the choice I made was myself rather than the role."

"Did you lose a sense of self or were you trying to recover it?"

"Had I ever had it? I was losing me as a priest but trying desperately to recover just me, James. Yes, this is a new thought. Perhaps I had spent my life as someone else in order not to be me."

"That thought sounds quite valuable."

"Yes, to explore what being me is. Me is something I see in the mirror. I have always had a difficulty with mirrors and photographs. I don't like being confronted by me."

"But the 'me' you see is not the 'me' that you are."

"No. That's true. But even in a mirror it's an image, a partial image. I don't want to but I have to look in a mirror, and apart from shaving I never do. I avoid them, and photographs. I find this much easier today than I ever did previously. I didn't like to have my photograph taken but then again, in this role as a curate or a vicar folk say, 'Well let's have a photograph,' after a baptism or a wedding, and you do it. And you say, 'Well, that's not me, that's the vicar.'"

"Diane Williams, a nurse, who has written in the States about having Möbius, said that initially she didn't know what was wrong. Then, as a nurse, she found a name for it and once she had a name she found it easier to talk to her friends about it. Once she talked, the face became a smaller part of what she was. Her self became more important and she was able then to confront the problem. As a young girl, however, a very important part of what she was, was this face. At that time though, paradoxically, she could only cope with it by putting it to one side."

"Yes, there's a very strong echo there with me. But it happened to me later. You see I have spent a lot of my life not being able to confront it, hiding behind a dog collar. Any development that has taken place more recently came about, in part, through the Möbius support group and seeing that there are other folk and other families that have it much worse and have had to struggle much harder than me. Though I think I had to struggle very hard, and have had to recently in deciding to think about these things more than I have done previously.

"My deciding to retire was not a loss of faith at all, quite the opposite. I no longer wanted to continue in the parochial ministry, but unfortunately there are not many nonparochial openings for clergymen. The counselor impressed on me that I could take charge of my life. I could decide things for myself, that I could make a choice and others would listen.

"They couldn't find a nonparochial position. In the end the bishop suggested medical retirement. A psychiatrist called it a chronic stress disorder and that was accepted by the Pensions' Board of the Church of England. At first I thought, well, I'm not a medical problem, I'm a spiritual problem, but then I thought that that's just a matter of pride, isn't it? After most of my life being a vicar or a priest, I wanted to be me. Now I want to find out what this means. I think I am beginning to feel much freer about myself, having made contact with that group.

"It is easier now to talk about myself. I had never previously talked to anyone very much. I love the Church of England and there are fine men among its leaders, but they don't really want to know. They may ask you how you are and it's OK if you say, 'Very well,' but if you say, 'I'm about to drop this tea tray,' they don't know what to do. Or they give you the impression that they'd say, 'Well, drop it, and then we can do something. But before then we're powerless.' I did go through a period in the late eighties when I was quite desperate and I would describe it in terms of 'I am going to drop this tea tray.' Perhaps to get attention, but I didn't really want to drop it, I just wanted someone to listen and do something. Those problems I didn't explicitly relate to the problems of the Möbius syndrome. But they do relate to the more general need to find myself, which in turn relates to the Möbius."

"Adolescence is a time to go out into the world, to learn to relate to others and to learn about yourself."

"Yes, I don't think I did that then. Perhaps I did turn my back on self-expression. Perhaps self-expression was beyond me. It was just quite enough to get by day to day. Meeting the Möbius group has had a good, very positive effect on me. I was fifty-three then and I had never even heard the name Möbius. It had never really occurred to me, nor had I wondered, consciously, how many like me are there out there."

"Film stars, models, and royal princesses live their lives around their faces to an extent. You seem to be saying that for much of your life you got by without it."

"Are you suggesting that I turned my back on my face? I don't know; I hadn't thought of it but I certainly may have done that, much more than I had ever realized or supposed. This idea I mentioned earlier of attempting to live behind it may well be an escape from something I found intolerable. By the time I was trying to decide whether to go or not to the meeting of the Möbius group I'd retired. I wondered whether I'd got beyond it but then I decided I would go and it would be part of finding out more about myself. I think I decided to go because I thought, well, I have survived. I thought if I go I will be one of the older ones and maybe other folk may realize that, however difficult things are now for them, for the youngsters, it is possible to survive, to go on. To some extent I feel I went for others."

"That's certainly how they saw you. They were delighted to have a mature and successful person who could act as some sort of role model."

"I also learned then that some folk are much more severely affected than others. It comes back a little to my upbringing. I think it was good that the family treated me no differently, treated me entirely normally. But I now realize that some things which may have been due to the condition I felt were just down to me. Rather than saying that the condition has made life difficult I have been saying, 'I have made life difficult. It was *my* fault. I have failed.' I think I was not coping with the job because I've not really faced up to myself. I think I have avoided reconciling myself to my problem."

"Maybe to become a whole person you had to look in the mirror, you had to say 'This is my face but I am not this: I exist behind and yet beyond it.'"

"Yes, I think you're right. One of the things I think that's happening now is that I have a sense of becoming freer. Freer in the sense of becoming more myself, not playing a role. I certainly wanted to try and explore me behind the mask of the priesthood. If you say where does 'me' now reside, I think I am slowly coming out of my head a bit. I am not sure I can locate where I am, but I don't think I am entirely in my head, or even my mind. I have an expression of living 'a life of the mind,' but I do accept that the mind is not easily able to communicate its thoughts or even its feelings. I think I was out of touch with my feelings, or I suppressed a lot of them. I have been told I am a very placid person. My sister said 'You never cried, you were a very good child in that sense.' I had all these things, operations, manipulations, splints, but I can't know now how much was a placidness of nature and how much was a suppression of feeling."

"But it was very difficult for you to express emotions physically, to make 'feelings.'"

"The lack of the smile is a scourge in the teenage years and is more of a problem than anything else, more than the eating in public. Being misunderstood, not being able to register recognition or salutation, and particularly with girls. If you look as though you don't know the girl, then she won't respond to you, will she? It is only recently that I came across the idea of nonverbal communication and that one can use one's hand as a way of showing recognition and of greeting someone. Before, I used to keep them by my side or fold them. They were just tools, not signals, until recently. Starting work, thirty years ago, when walking along a street, I didn't sneak along by the side of the houses, but I was very defensive in the way I went about. I don't now wear a clerical collar during the week because I want to be me rather than someone holding an office. I did find it awkward walking around in uniform, I felt even more conspicuous, whereas today I don't care. If they say, 'Hello,' I'll say, 'Hello,' or even I will say, 'Hello' first. I'm getting there."

"We've discussed your sense of self, and where you feel it resides, and you seem to be saying that more and more it resides in your body, in your arms, rather than just in your head. The further you are in your body the closer you are to the world."

"Yes. I think that's so."

"How do you view other people's faces?"

"I used to be accused of staring at people long ago and of course I have to turn the head, because I can't turn the eyes, in order to look at people, and there's not much movement of the face, so youngsters used to say, 'Who are you staring at?' So perhaps because of this I didn't look at people. One of my brothers has recently said that I am now looking at him more than I used to, so that's a good thing."

"I can't imagine a certain transient happiness without smiling. Have you ever felt it is more difficult to experience extreme happiness or sadness or even less obvious transient moods like this, or have you just dissociated the way in which you view moods from any bodily expression of them?"

"I think there's a lot of dissociation. But I do think I get trapped in my mind or my head. I sort of *think* happy or I *think* sad, not really saying or recognizing actually feeling happy or feeling sad. Perhaps I have had a difficulty in recognizing that which I'm putting a name to is not a thought at all but it is a feeling. Maybe I have to intellectualize mood. I have to say this thought is a happy thought, and therefore I am happy.

"I think also that I have a fear of being out of control with emotions, feeling something that I can't manage. I have also found it very difficult to communicate feelings throughout my life, whether as a child or with my wife, though I think I am getting better at it now. I don't really know how I communicate happiness or sadness. That's a very hard question. Some people cry when they're sad. I don't think I cry. I sometimes felt that I would like to be able to cry but you see I am not really able to cry, my tears can come but there's nothing else. My tears only flow when I eat. I am afraid of such feelings. I try and shut them off."

"The 'feeling' of sadness encompasses, in most people's parlance, both an internal state and a movement in the face. You are unable to experience the "external" feeling of sadness where it is on the face."

"When there are things which are sad I tell the person that I feel very sorry for you but I'm thinking that rather than feeling it. Of course, since I have never been able to move the face, I've never associated movement of the face with feeling of an emotion. If I have expressed any emotion I must have spoken it or I might put my arm around someone of course. Coming back to my job, however, I am not required to feel what I am trying to express."

"When you see a very funny program on the television and there's canned laughter, do you enter into that?"

"If I think it's funny, I think I do laugh, but I don't laugh a lot."

"Because you haven't been able to reinforce the feeling by laughter, you may not have experienced the feeling inside as much?"

"Yes, I think that's so. I think you're right. Those feelings are there but they're probably reduced."

"Disconnection may reduce involvement."

"Yes, I've often thought of myself as a spectator rather than as a participant."

"As the vicar you might have been described as a professional spectator."

"Yes."

"Maybe in leaving the parochial ministry you are discovering your true nonspectator self and in order to do that you have had to confront the Möbius and say, 'I have this problem but I am not any different from anyone else behind it.'"

"Yes, but people: they are their faces. I think I would like to be my face. I am beginning to want to be my face. Possibly like the black who's initially black and ashamed but then becomes black and proud. I may become more assertive without being more aggressive. In the past I have often had an idea but not managed to do something, whereas now I am beginning to do something, whether its the idea to ring someone up or send them a card, I actually follow it through. I am becoming more proactive. I am entering into the world more than in the past."

"In Exodus Moses was not allowed to see the face of God, though he could see his back. Why?"

"Because its too much, too intense, too bright. I don't really know why you can't see the face. There's no description of Christ in the New Testament. But it's not peculiar to Christ; there's no description of others."

"The Lord brings his face to shine upon you."

"Yes, that's one of the great blessings. It's a poetic image. I can read faces but I can't give a face in return. In that sense I am invisible or blank. I may have traded on the blankness from time to time. I have sometimes thought, when I have felt low, if only other people knew what I am thinking. Other people may not want to have thoughts that they're feeling portrayed to others. I know that none of my thoughts will ever be seen by others on my face."

I went out to the toilet feeling thoughts and thinking feelings, ideas about the relation of feelings to their communication chasing around in my head. When I returned James was reading his Bible.

"I was looking at a passage in Isaiah, said to relate to Christ, Isaiah 53: beginning verse 2:

He had no beauty, no majesty to draw our eyes,
No grace to make us delight in him;
His form, disfigured, lost all the likeness of a man, his
beauty changed beyond human semblance.
He was despised, he shrank from the sight of men,
tormented and humbled by suffering;
We despised him. We held him of no account, the
thing from which men turn away their eyes.
He was afflicted, . . . and did not open his mouth . . .
He was cut off from the world of living men."

"It's only in more recent times that I've dared to think of that passage in terms of myself. I could not obviously claim all of that, but I do feel that I fit in somewhere. What I would say is that several years ago I would never have thought of seeing myself there and if I had, I'd have thought, that's wrong, that's blasphemous. But now I think I understand those words better and they have a personal involvement for me and they have a message, which is, 'This is how I am and I must accept it, can accept it,' and in being related to me they are very positive words too. I have never used in a sermon or an address anything personal or about my situation in talking to people. One day I might have the confidence to do that. Or find circumstances in which it might be appropriate to raise it."

"Surely one reason Christ came on Earth was not to expropriate suffering into the divine but to show us that suffering was part of the human condition, and understood as such by God. What use is the Bible if it does not allow us to consider our suffering? Surely it is not blasphemous to think of one's suffering in the same terms as those used in the Bible?

"In the past I wouldn't have put my face or my experiences with this, but it does have a place in that context. I see that now, much more clearly. Thirty years ago I didn't, it was inappropriate, it was a denial. I was denying the face. My face. I think I am beginning to feel that I can think that way, realize my face, and almost in some way be glad of it or accept it. I had lost the sense that God was my Father, but slowly I am regaining that. A counselor priest asked me how I viewed myself in relation to God, and this set me thinking. I am slowly realizing that I can be His son. I can be worthy, and worthy without having to try to be so. I am beginning to realize that we don't have to try to be worthy, that worthiness or love is absolute and unconditional, an acceptance, and this I think is also very relevant for the way we approach others and those we love. It's ironic that I left the Church in terms of the parochial ministry to discover this."

After tea as I drove away, James was waving. Not much, but more than maybe he had done for most of his life. He had told me of things he had previously not discussed with anyone, and by their telling had maybe explored them more than he had done previously. I felt humbled and overawed by his personal new testament.

One Big Family

James's priestly witness had shown me a rich and moving life lived without a mobile expressive face. Yet I was uncertain if his story was typical. Though his witness had relevance regardless of others' experiences, I wanted to know something of others with Möbius syndrome.

I also wanted to see some children with the condition together. Some years ago children with Möbius were thought to be autistic because they had severe problems in socializing with others. Assuming such children had no coexistent autism, their problems in social development and self-awareness seemed to arise out of, and originate in, their facial problems. I wanted to see a group of these children at play. Would they squabble and fight and form friends and gangs like children in any noisy playground, or would they be more quiet, isolated and detached from their peers?

Recently in the UK, as James revealed, there has been set up a support group for those with Möbius syndrome and their families. (There is now also a group in the US.) I went to their summer meeting in a seaside town on the east coast, expecting to listen and observe. I arrived at the hotel the night before and, after a run, spent the evening on the beach, watching the people walking up and down. Most were enjoying the late sun and their time together. Families and lovers were smiling, laughing, chatting about anything and nothing—the words were irrelevant, their faces were telling the more important stories of feelings and mood.

The next morning the meeting began with introductions. Persons with Möbius or their parents stood up to introduce themselves. There were about fifteen to twenty persons with the condition, mostly young children but also teenagers and adults. In my short talk I told the audience how my interest had been aroused by Mary, and how most doctor friends had little professional awareness of facial expression and of its importance. I gave a resume of ideas about the face's importance in the expression of emotion and even, possibly, for its experience.

Prompted by my talk, Jane Walker, a senior orthoptist from Great Ormond Street, who has treated more than forty people with Möbius over nearly thirty years, told of some research in which a clinical psychologist had given children with the syndrome a series of photographs of faces and asked them what the person's feelings were from their facial expressions. The children were almost completely unable to interpret the feelings of others from such photos. This surprised some of the parents, several of whom spoke of their children having no problem in either expressing themselves, nor apparently in tuning in to others.

Next, Robert, a twenty-two-year-old student, stood up and with a beautifully dry sense of humor, and considerable courage, conveyed a life.

"When I heard about the Möbius support group I thought, 'shock, horror,' there are other people like me. So I thought I'd come down and tell you something of my life.

"When I was born the doctor said I wouldn't live. I didn't learn to speak until I was five. When I was little I used to have a fascination with cars and consequently my first word was Renault.

"I went to a succession of special schools. They were wonderful to me though other people may have different feelings. Mine were a delight. Unfortunately, when I went to comprehensive school, at fourteen, I learned that it was all about holding one's head up above the water and trying not to get clattered [beaten] by the local toughs. I was getting roughed up by some of the bullies who were a lot bigger than me. Once when I got hit by one of the bullies I hit him back quite hard; after that the bullies didn't bully so much and the school was very happy I'd done it too. I was very pleased too; it was quite an experience. After I left school I went to Hereward College [an extended education college for the disabled]. They treated you like a human being, admittedly with difficulties, but nevertheless a human being. I took further GCSEs [General Certificate of Secondary Education] and then I decided to go to the local college where I took several A levels.

"By then I was twenty-one and I was thinking, what do I want to do with the rest of my life? I was obviously not going to be a male model but I had always had a desire to do journalism. I found a place and the local council were very good at supporting my education and helping me with accommodation. I found a flat—after a term I decided it would be nice to have my own house and I got together with three friends and we now rent out a place together. Living together is quite fun as long as we all do the washing up. We all get up together, we wash up together, and we get drunk together. It's only when you're living in a house like that that you understand what independence means. I have the attic room and I can see miles over the hills so I'm quite enjoying myself.

"Not long ago there was a student competition in journalism—you had to write an essay on what the role of student newspapers was. Well, I won a trip to Los Angeles. To think, not long ago I was concerned about going out at all and now I'm off to America. The point is, that when I was at my special school I never thought I would do anything. I thought I'd live with my mum and dad for ever. If you set your sights high enough, though they have to be realistic goals, then I reckon you can do it. Anyone who's disabled, my message is, Go and achieve what you want. There's no one going to stop you but yourself."

He delivered this without notes, with a mastery of timing and humor. The whole audience warmed to him and the Möbius syndrome melted away. He was just Rob, jokes and all.

There was a long lunch break and I sat talking with Clare and her parents. She had known of my coming for some time and had agreed to talk with me. Clare was in her early thirties. I had noticed her sitting in the main group earlier, though it was her mother who had stood up at the introduction. I began by asking her mother about Clare's childhood.

"When she was born she couldn't suck. We tried everything to get her to feed, from small spoons to premature baby feeders and in the end we used a soft teat. When she was eight months we took her to Great Ormond Street where they made the diagnosis but didn't give us much indication as to what that would mean. Her father took her and asked

'Do you think she is backward?' and the doctor said 'No, she's just a bit behind."[1] She was very slow in her milestones—she didn't speak really until she went to school and she went to an educationally subnormal school, [now called a school for those with learning difficulties]. Nobody really knows why she didn't speak. We don't think she should have gone to the ESN school. If she could have coped with the mainstream school because of her face, she'd have certainly coped because of her intellect.

"She's always been very highly strung. If she was sitting down or in a pram and I'd walk out of the room she'd scream. She screamed a lot. At the hospital they said she was frustrated. She would have a go at her elder sisters. If I didn't take her with me everywhere then she'd scream; if I went upstairs at all she had to come with me—she went everywhere with me.

"We didn't have a night's sleep for four years; she used to scream and wake us up. Thinking back, I realize it was because she couldn't shut her eyes. She may have just woken up and been frightened of the dark and she couldn't shut her eyes. Maybe if we'd had a small light or if we'd had her in with us it may have been better. To wake up in the pitch black and be unable to see anything must have been terrifying."

If she did not talk until she was five or so I wondered what was going on in her mind.

"I imagine she thought a lot, I don't know. When I was in the room she followed me with her eyes and her head of course, but as soon as I left the room she'd yell out. They worked her into school very gradually, initially in the morning, then for a bit longer, and then a whole day, and then I would leave. Initially she would scream the place down continually and eventually they said 'Don't take any notice, just go' and then when I left her there at lunchtime the first day she was perfectly OK and for the rest of her time there she was fine. She didn't have any of her temper tantrums for the duration of her time at school. It gave her something to do.

"Now she feels rather cheated because life has passed her by. She reads in church and she gives Communion. She could have done more. At this stage of her life she is frustrated. She sees her sisters getting on and she hasn't. She goes to a day center just for something to do and they do various projects. Her friends are all older people, both in church and at the day center."

Clare was sitting next to me, and I had been addressing her mother across the room, trying to make sure my questions were suitable. I was a little surprised by some of her mother's replies, though Clare seemed fascinated and almost relieved to have such matters aired. But she did not interrupt. Then, in answer to a direct question, she started to speak.

"My first childhood memory is of having my teeth out at three. A big black mask came over my face. Even now if somebody goes toward me I can't bear it."

Try to imagine having a mask come down and be unable to look away or to close your eyes as an understanding adult, and now as a child. Her mother took it up again.

"In really stressed situations she'd lose control. She couldn't cope any more and this would manifest itself by falling down, kicking out, spluttering, shouting, lying there. Once she ended up in casualty. She's had two EEGs to try and establish whether these episodes are epileptic or not. Earlier in the year she had a severe episode. She was at home with her father because I was in hospital. Everything got on top of her. She'd actually been in psychiatric hospitals because of her emotional outbursts in the past and had once ended up in a straitjacket. On this occasion, however, she walked round to the GP [general practitioner] and asked to go to the local psychiatric hospital. An amazingly controlled thing to do—an emotional outburst which involved walking three quarters of a mile to a GP's surgery. Her father went up to the GP's surgery and she refused to go home. She was admitted to the hospital overnight and then stayed with her sister for a few weeks."

I asked what an attack was like. Clare laughed, the small high laugh I had soon learned to interpret in various ways in response to my questions. She still looked across at her mother. "Well," her mother said to Clare, "Are you telling me you can't remember what its like?"

Clare replied, "But I do remember. Although I try and block it out of my mind. I know what's going on. Its like, I suppose, as Sheila says 'It's like a tantrum,' but I can't cope with assertive situations."

I suggested that we might say something's awful, or bloody awful, but that she found it difficult, even impossible, to express emotions until they boil over. "With people who you don't know, and who are unaware of what you are thinking or feeling, you might go from nothing to a meltdown?"

"That's fair. Yeah."

Her mother came in, "Maybe that's why priests have breakdowns 'cos they can't express emotion either."

Clare spoke,

"I've always felt it difficult to express how I feel. I know its only in the last couple of years that, say, at church when I meet someone I just say 'I can't smile' and then it becomes easier. For thirty years or so I used to put it to the back of my mind. It didn't worry me and now I'm beginning to be more aware of it."

I continued, "Did you ever feel as James did [she knew James from a previous meeting] that the up and down part of your emotional states were different to others?"

"Not when I was young. But it is happening now. When I was younger I didn't know, I just accepted that that's how I was."

"James said he has to think that he's smiling or happy, rather than actually feel happy."

"Yes, I feel that too. The spontaneity of feeling isn't as acute."

By now Clare felt able to initiate conversation. "I first met someone else with the Möbius two years ago at the meeting. It was wonderful. We sat in the hotel and we knew there was another one coming in, and then another one, and then another one, and initially we were all a bit shy but by the next day we were talking to each other, swapping experiences. Because we all look the same its like one big family.[2] I felt well . . . [a long pause] . . . happy, really happy."

"Do you remember getting excited at Christmas or birthdays?"

"Not really."

Mother again.

"She was very quiet. For many years she would only go out with her sister or her parents. Sheila used to go to the nearest town with her. By the time Clare was twenty they'd stand at a bus stop. Sheila would get on the first bus and wait at the other end and Clare would get on the next one so that she would at least be on the bus on her own. The idea of getting a train, say to London on her own, is not one she could contemplate."

I finally raised the obvious, that when I asked a question, looking at Clare, she would laugh and not say anything and then look across at her mother for the answer.

"I know. Its like that. When Mum's here it's . . . I talk and she answers and when she's not here I'm much better."

"Perhaps I should go into the garden with you, without your mother. What do you think?"

"I don't know."

A little while later Clare suggested to her mother that we might be left on our own for a few minutes. I had the feeling that this took quite a lot for her to ask. We sat for some time in the quiet, I had no need to talk, and she was perhaps searching, not for what to say, but for the right weight and words to use.

"I love my parents but they're overprotective. Also I lack confidence. OK, I'm talking to you now but I was very nervous about your coming."

I reassured her that I too was nervous about the visit. I asked if most of her friends were at church, so they may have known her since she was born.

"My father was a Catholic but my mother and I only became Catholics about ten years ago and have only been in that church for that length of time."

"Then it must have taken a lot of courage for you to go into somewhere you weren't known?"

"It did. I don't know a way of getting round the face problem in meeting people. With time, as I get to know people, then it becomes easier. I've now taken to telling them. For instance, I recently went to a new hairdresser's. She was smiling and engaging me in conversation and in the end I just had to tell her that I couldn't smile. I feel better when I've told someone."

"When you're sad, how do you tell someone that you're sad?"

"Mm, well, I don't—I can't. I think I've always been aware of such problems. At a wedding recently the photographer kept saying 'well, smile' to everyone and I had to say 'I can't smile.' Maybe I couldn't have been so forthright a few years ago."

"How do you tell someone when you're feeling good?"

"I don't."

"Do you use body language much? Might it help?"

"I think I do use it, say at church. I recently leant over and touched someone. I may not have done that a few years ago. To wave back, even to someone I know, requires confidence and for a long time, perhaps, I wouldn't have done that because I lack the assertiveness or I was shy. I remember that I used to get upset on my mother's behalf, and I still do, that people were staring at me and how she must feel. I very rarely went out when I was younger. Looking back, I wish I'd had more of an independent life. I really did enjoy being a care assistant. I enjoyed feeding the old people and I think they liked me 'cos they gave me an eighteenth birthday present, some china figures and a record."

I returned to her attacks and asked if she had any warning.

"Yeah, I know, for several minutes. Often I wake up feeling sad, or bad, and it's building up inside me and I know it's going to happen and things progress. Though my mother doesn't realize it, I do know what I'm doing. I don't think people know how tense I am. It is very frustrating when no one knows how worked up I am. Its better now because I've found ways of telling them. At church I used to read, but I've stopped doing that—it made me too nervous. Now I actually give the sacrament of Communion. I go to various places and actually stand there and do it. A lot of people say they couldn't do it, they'd have to stand up in front of other people. It is quite daunting but I want to do it."

"Do you feel that you observe life rather than take part in it? Might it be better if you could initiate things?"

"Yes. Exactly. Yes. That's it. Yes, that's very fair. If someone said 'Tell me what you want,' I wouldn't know because I haven't sampled it."

I was unsure if I was putting questions into her mouth, or if she was telling of things she had often thought of but never dared say. "Is it fair to suggest that your inability to express various emotions, not just happiness or sadness—those are just extremes—all the different emotions, means that people think of you in the passive."

"Yes, that's right. I haven't had those experiences. I just want to take part."

"I hope you're agreeing because it is right, not just because I'm saying it."

"No, you seem to understand."

"Is there a part of you that accepts that if you were able to express emotion more you would be able to experience emotion better?"

"Yes, I know what you mean."

"It's not only that you find it more difficult to communicate emotion but that you actually find it more difficult to experience it yourself."

"Yes, I feel that."

Her sister Sheila appeared to see how we were getting on and to give Clare a rest. She suggested that but for the Möbius Clare would have been like her, shy to start with, but then very outgoing and fun once among friends. She had grown up with her sister and knew Clare better than anyone. I thanked Clare for talking. She thanked me. She liked deep things, she said. I had the same feeling as when I had left James. Both, having known for some time ahead that I was coming, had decided to talk about their lives in a way they had never done previously. I had the small hope that through talking about their problems they may have understood them a little better. Both had been "priestly witnesses," both in John Hull's term, and in finding in ritual and religion a sense of self and of purpose not available elsewhere.

In the afternoon there were no organized talks and we were free to wander between rooms. One of the children there was Duncan, an eight-year-old boy I had met some months earlier. At that time I had gone to talk with him and his parents. Duncan, faced with a stranger and after a day's school, had gone to play outside. So I sat with his mother.

"My other children had been precocious, smiling, sitting, standing earlier than most other children, but with Duncan it was quite the reverse. I looked on him as a real baby, and did not dislike it. Even then there were odd things, for instance, the other children recognized me when I went in the room: Duncan's never done that. Then suddenly I realized that he was no longer a baby and yet was still not doing things. By eight months people were whispering that something was wrong with him. My other children had been smiling and crawling around by then, but Duncan didn't do anything. He was a very cuddly baby but he never returned the smiles. The first time I really understood what was going on inside his head was one day when I was looking for a nappy pin for my youngest and he said, 'Me get it,' and he went and fetched it from the drawer. He was three then. Up until then no one had known what intelligence Duncan might have. He had been completely passive, seeing and hearing, but unable to impose a sound or thought or emotion upon those around him."

Fortunately, the problems were picked up and he went to a special school early—he couldn't talk until he was about three and a half—and improved enormously with physiotherapy and speech therapy. He had a one-on-one helper for twenty five hours a week teaching him and helping him with the hand and speech problems as well as with the learning disability. At the school all he wanted was a wheelchair so that he could go abseiling down walls like the other kids. He soon learned that Möbius was not only a handicap. Sometimes he would bully smaller boys. Because he is such an innocent appearing boy and doesn't show emotion, people don't think he's capable of various things. No one could tell whether he's lying or not. You had to actually catch him. What is also apparent was the way in which, because he did not invest meaning into his face, he regarded it less and cared for it less than other children and adults.

"He just sits there like a little stuffed dummy—he doesn't touch his face in a gestural manner.[3] We had to teach him to feel his face because he was dribbling. Now we've taught him, Duncan does play with his face and feel it, but still mainly to see if it is wet."

In place of the spontaneous volcanic emotions children experience, display, and learn to control, Duncan, like Clare, inhabits a rather isolated world of deliberation and thought.

"Once, after his brothers had been unkind, he waited until they went out to play and then he went upstairs to their bedroom and smeared toothpaste all over the inside of their beds. We smelt something for a long time but it was only in the evening that we realized what he'd done. He really thinks about what he does and he never does the obvious thing. For instance, he hides things to torment people; one shoe for instance. He thinks about things far more before he does them than our other children. He's often off in his own little world working out what to do. He can sit up all night, till 3 or 4 o'clock in the morning and he'll pop down and eat something in the cupboard. We don't know what's going on in his head. He's too busy to sleep."

The highlights of a normal childhood seemed to pass him by too.

"I remember his fifth birthday party. He was sat in his highchair and went to sleep. It was just like another day for him. He didn't want to know, he didn't want to play. He doesn't really get excited on birthdays, even his own; it's just like another day to him. It is difficult to know when he's having fun. When he comes home from school we don't know how he's feeling, we have to ask him. Everything is questions and answers. He has always been a very placid child. He never really gets angry, never really gets upset. One thing that does upset him is a lack of friends at school. He will go upstairs and sulk and make his cry, which is more of a whine, and when he feels better he'll come down. His lip does come out a little bit when he's upset."

Though his parents have talked little about the Möbius to him, there is no doubt that Duncan is aware. Not long ago he came rushing into the bathroom to his mother and said "It has moved, it has moved." He was so excited, "My eyes moved." His mother continued, "I wish with Duncan I had taken more photographs. Because he never did anything and you usually take milestones, I never took them. He always sits back and listens and stores things for later, much more reflective. We always cuddle him but it's true that probably, because he's so thoughtful and reflective, our approach to him is less spontaneous. I used to cuddle him but he never really cuddled back. Now I still cuddle him because he's my baby, but he just sits there saying 'I'm too old for this now, Mum.'"

When I saw him at the meeting six months later the improvement in facial movement was obvious; Duncan was trudging around taking everything in, with a quizzical Duncan-style face. He even walked up, hands in pockets, and said "Hi, Jonathan" and smiled. Smiled with his body and his voice, but also a little around the eyes and with his face. I was thrilled to be approached and we talked. He was clearly bright and intelligent with a wicked sense of humor, and his Möbius was not as severe as some. I hoped he might catch up, even at his early age. I thought he would.

George

Later I spoke with George, who happened to be over from Canada for the summer and had come along somewhat reluctantly. His grandmother has a tape of him reciting and singing when he was two. He is now a poet who often appears at public readings.

George is an obviously handsome man, outgoing in his gestures and in his voice, a person whose presence fires a room. There's a musicality in his voice which makes one attend to it, and to him. His Möbius seems almost an irrelevance. I asked if he had ever consciously decided to use body language more.

"Yes, I think I did, though I can't remember exactly when. It's odd but occasionally friends will say that they just don't know what I'm feeling, or what I'm about to do. As I've got older I try to give people more clues as to what I'm doing or what I'm feeling in my mannerisms, in my body language, and in my voice, in everything I have. I try and use everything I've got. I do more. I don't think about my face at all—it's only when I have to meet new people. Then its always in the back of my mind that I'll have to tell someone new about my problem and I have to speak slightly differently."

Later he did a short reading, the sound of which filled the hall. Parents and grandparents of young people with Möbius were just in awe. I thought of John Hull and Peter White saying that their character resides in their voice. George's voice proclaimed someone not simply managing to exist but a person with such exuberance and beauty as to leave most other people behind. That he could do this and proclaim his character in such a way was a simple, miraculous inspiration.

Yet there was a problem. He was an individual and just wanted to be known for what he was, like anyone else. My concentration, and the day's concentration on Möbius, annoyed him. Why couldn't I just accept him, and not ask questions? I felt mean, for though I was interested in the illness, my interest was not in the disease itself but in its effects on individuals. I had not come to the meeting as a doctor, but as a person trying to understand how individuality develops with Möbius, how it can be lived with and yet overcome.

What if Möbius children had grown up in a world of the blind? They would have been able to help their friends around. Would their emotional lives then have been like their unsighted brothers and sisters? These were some of the intellectual ideas I was asking. The other, human questions of how to help those present, and of the whole approach to disability, were impressing themselves on me in scarcely delineated ways. How might we pass on experience from one generation with Möbius to the next? That was what the day was for, and that, despite George, required concentration on the syndrome. Though detesting the day, he agreed on that question and has found his own answer by helping the parents of a young child with Möbius.

Several of the parents sought me out. They didn't think they had difficulty in understanding what their sons and daughters were feeling or wanting to express. Even with small movements of a lip or a little movement around the eyes they had learned to interpret these as expressions of various moods. I still had some concerns. These children were preschool children, who had only known a loving family life. What would happen when they entered school and had to meet new people? One mother came up to me and said that her young boy was very able to make himself understood within the family, but when he went outside to play the other children didn't take much notice of him.

I was anxious to spend sometime with the dozen or so children in their crèche. In a corner a large TV was showing Disney videos—few of the children took any notice and I turned over to the cricket for a short while. Instead the children were sitting on their own, playing with Lego and other games, or were being read to by parents and carers. There were few of the interactions and new friendships that young children usually make, and the room was quiet, quiet in a way I had not known a room full of kids to be before. Maybe I was bringing my preconceptions with me, but there seemed less seeking out of other children than I was used to seeing at schools and parties. It was not just that the children did not know one another, they showed little inclination to make a move toward others. Maybe this was why they had been thought autistic in the past.

It was clear, however, from the day that the stories of James and of Clare were not typical, for many of the people with Möbius there were doing well in their lives. A few years ago Jane Walker had sent a questionnaire out to persons with Möbius. The questions were very hard emotionally. That she was able to ask them reflects her knowledge of, and love for, the people she was looking after, and the affection and respect they hold her in. She asked parents and guardians of the youngest group how they felt when they first knew that their child would be unable to express emotion and how the child expressed his or her feelings. Teenagers were asked about difficulties in meeting people and if more facial expression would have made it easier to get along with others; if they were happier, more depressed, or were aggressive than their peers. Adults were asked whether they were happy with their appearance at work and socially.

The answers were overwhelmingly positive. Most people felt that they had overcome the problems. One wrote that she never gave the

Möbius a thought. They were, on the whole, happy with whom they had become. Only one out of the twenty responders did not have a good or reasonably good social interaction. It is not clear why some succeed and others fail: perhaps the syndrome is more severe in some, perhaps the way in which parents and loved ones respond to the child affects development. Much is unknown.

I left the weekend as the children went off to a local amusement park. One person, who had cared for many people with Möbius over three decades, told me that she found it more difficult to understand the condition than deafness or blindness. Yet the very fact that people with Möbius had so many different experiences renewed my faith in people's abilities to find ways around medical and developmental problems, and to do so in ways that allowed and enabled individuality.

Yet despite this I came back again and again to James. James, courageously, in his fifties, was beginning to explore who he was and to accept his face, having for years existed despite it. His experience might not be typical, but he seemed to have taken matters further than the others, having lived with Möbius longer than most. His reflections seemed somehow important not just for his development, but also for the way in which the face normally enables expression and expression aids selfhood. Duncan's and Clare's lack of emotional highs at birthdays, and their introspection, seemed linked to James's experience. It was as though the displaying of emotion on the face enabled its full feeling and expression within, as William James had intimated. Without the ability to show to others, a full social existence was scarcely possible, and without these relationships the inner feelings could not develop.

One man with Möbius and in his twenties had not come to the meeting but instead had written describing his outward success as a teacher. Privately, however, he was deeply depressed by his condition. It was all made worse by the façade he was expected to display to everyone in both his professional and personal life. Eventually, he had broken down, unable to carry the weight of his denial, like James unable to maintain his façade over a lifetime. After a period in hospital he had become able to accept Möbius and to exist with it and despite it. He had written his story to alert others, to have them not ignore it but confront it, and then live with it. "Help each other," he wrote, "your experiences are unique."

James wrote to me subsequently and reiterated that he had not talked about his face before. It had been a new idea to him that his difficulties in life were related directly to the face rather than to him in general. His family, by treating him normally in his first few years, were acting out of the best of all motives and gave him an enchanted start. But by not exploring the facial problem they may have led James to ignore it as a source of his later difficulties, difficulties which after five decades he is now beginning to explore. Reading a draft of his conversation James had been surprised by the force with which he expressed himself, suggesting that his language may have had to carry something of what is lost without nonverbal communication.[4]

I was very reticent about exploring these personal details in conversation with both James and Clare, but they both, independently, approached our meetings as a chance to explore their feelings in a way they had not previously done. Clare, for instance, wrote that my visit had been the first time in her life that she had been able to express her feelings, and so gain some insight into herself.

James and Clare found themselves withdrawing from much social intercourse because they could not take part fully. The impassivity of their features may have reduced their sense of ownership of themselves and their emotions, and it may have reduced those feelings themselves.[5] But it also prevented any graded outlet for feelings they did have. James talked of "a fear of being out of control, feeling something I can't manage." Clare's losses of control were clearly when she could no longer contain herself and yet could not express her feelings—except by orchestrated tantrums. Möbius seems not only to dull the experience of some emotions but also lead to a fear of the great emotions that can rise up and explode uncontrollably. Perhaps it is through their expression that we normally learn about anger and grief and many other emotions and their acceptability for ourselves and others. James suggested that he may have been slow to recognize his feelings, slow to identify them as such, translating them into ideas and articulating them as thoughts. On reflection, he wrote, there may have been a gap between inner feeling and physical expression because of the face, thus explaining why, in his conversation, "I think" and "I feel" were interchangeable.[6]

I thought how we all as children gain some sort of understanding of the world and of ourselves. What sets us apart from other animals is not simply speech, hands, or tools, but an emotional complexity that is not only reflected and paralleled in our facial mobility but which is crucially dependent on it for communication and, perhaps, for full expression and development as an individual. Those with Möbius had much to teach us about the face. James ended a letter to me:

I do not really believe that anyone can live, or exist even, entirely inside his head. In terms of locating where my sense of myself presently resides, the idea does have meaning. I am sure that I have come out of my head quite a lot. Something you said struck me as important: "The further you are in your body, the closer you are to the world." I want to say "Amen," to that, and make it my aim for the future.

Dull and Boring?

Facial animation is congenitally absent in those with Möbius syndrome, but it can also be lost later in life in several other neurological conditions. The first case I had seen was Mary, whose story inspired me to look into the face. Her problem, though never confirmed, almost certainly involved strokes in part or parts of the brain, and she, unfortunately, never recovered.

One criticism never far from airing of first accounts is the inability of, say, someone congenitally blind to understand what it is like to see, though those of us who have sight are assumed to be able to understand what it is like to be blind. For blind, read autistic or Möbius. One of the important aspects of John Hull's account is that he has gone from one state, of seeing, to another, complete blindness. Equivalent transitions have not been described in autism or Möbius for obvious reasons (though some facial reanimation operations are being performed in Möbius subjects). There are, however, several other neurological causes of loss of facial animation with the possibility of recovery which might allow the two sides of this question to be addressed at firsthand.

Charles Bell described loss of function of one facial nerve leading to dropping of that side of the face, an illness still known as Bell's palsy: most people will have seen cases of this either in the street or among friends, and in most cases some recovery occurs. Though infrequent, there are cases in which both sides of the face are affected. Bell wrote that such a person's face is worse than that of a statue, for at least a statue has a single recognizable facial expression. I talked with two people with this condition, whose loss of facial movement had occurred suddenly and catastrophically. In Parkinson's disease, in contrast, loss of facial animation can occur insidiously and often is not noticed. These persons offer a different perspective on "losing face," for their lack of animation is often not realized, friends and relatives alike simply thinking that the person has become dull and boring.

I went to talk with some of these people, trying to uncover the differences between losing facial animation as an adult as opposed to never having had it, remembering how different congenital and acquired blindness were in this situation and, where recovery had occurred, to ask how this temporary period of facial immobility was viewed.

Oliver

After an undistinguished time at public school Oliver required a few terms at a London "crammer" college to pass his university entrance exams. He decided to follow his father into architecture. Since some of the more fashionable courses were beyond his reach, he ended up as the only southerner in Middlesborough, an unforgiving steel and chemical town in northeast England. He need not have worried, for he soon settled down, managing on the way to disabuse many of his new friends about southern softies.

It was just before Christmas of his final year that he woke up with conjunctivitis. Both eyes were completely bloodshot, so he made an appointment to see a doctor who diagnosed conjunctivitis and gave antibiotics. A couple of days later he and his friends left a house party and went off to a pub. It was then that he felt the left half of his face go "numb," a numbness which he soon realized meant it was paralyzed. "I put it down to the alcohol and ignored it all evening. It got worse—so I got drunker. The next day it was still there and I had a fright, but because the friends had come up for the weekend I didn't want to disappoint them. We went off to Newcastle for the day, forty miles away."

On the way he realized that he hadn't eaten since the previous lunchtime. They went to a McDonald's, which fortunately had seats in line with the table so he did not have to face anyone. Once back at the house, however, he could conceal it no longer and his roommate made him see a doctor. The casualty doctor diagnosed Bell's palsy and gave him steroids. Then Oliver went back to partying, after reassurance that alcohol would have no effect on the condition or on the tablets. The next day he watched a film in the afternoon, but his eyes were so bad that by the end he could hardly see a thing. He went to see his own doctor again, by now a week or so after the first appointment. His doctor agreed it was Bell's palsy and that the eyes would not clear up because of it. But Oliver knew that both eyes were affected, so what had the single-sided Bell's got to do with it?

That weekend he woke up with the right side of the face gone as well. He immediately saw another doctor who told him to come back in a week.

"By that stage I was beginning to panic. Up to that point I had not been too worried but when both sides no longer worked I was very scared. What was happening to my face? I could not go out on my own and had to ask one of my flat mates to go out with me. In fact I didn't want to go out and was taken by a friend down to the GP's. I always had someone with me to shop—I needed someone to be with me. I could not talk properly and it was awful not being able to communicate."

Losing confidence fast, he went to see his course leader, who suggested that he go home until next term. Once there, things moved more quickly. His parents arranged for him to be admitted to a hospital and over the next few days he had all sorts of checks, including a brain scan and an examination of the spinal fluid, as well as neurological observations every few hours, day and night.

There was a man on the ward who had just been told he had terminal cancer. On the last day he came and sat on Oliver's bed and told him about his illness. "I said how sorry I was. My mother was there and, when I went out of the room, she started talking to the man's wife. Because of my face the wife thought I had been totally unsympathetic to the man's problem."

He left the hospital after a few days, exhausted, and went next to see an ophthalmic surgeon who found inflammation of the inner eye, and thought it was sarcoid, so the steroids were continued.[1] There then followed several weeks at home, with little change in the face, though the eyes cleared up. It was then that I saw him.

As we talked Oliver covered the lower part of his face, lifting up the lower lip to close the mouth, which moved a very small amount.

The muscles around the eyes and the eyebrows were working more, but his face was still almost completely impassive, like Bell's original cases.

"Because I cannot see myself I forget what the problem is. And because I have some slight movement around the mouth that I can feel but which you cannot see, I look worse than I feel. Until I stand in front of a mirror and realize that I cannot smile it is not at the forefront of my mind. When I only had one side go I was sitting at a table. People on my left side would make a joke and I would laugh with my right face but not my left. People on my one side had no problem while those on my other thought I had gone awfully serious. It was weird, as though I was two people."

As in those with Möbius I had the impression that without facial animation Oliver's moods and feelings themselves were lessened. I asked how he felt, not just with the illness—that was obviously a cause for concern—but how he actually *felt,* with an immobile face.

"I suppose I don't feel constantly happy, but then I don't feel sad . . . I feel almost as if I am in a limbo between feelings—just non-emotional . . . I don't know . . . "

"But you are in a limbo of sorts, at home when you want to be doing the course, with your friends, getting on with life."

"Yes, but it is within myself, an emotional limbo. I still feel happy to see or hear something I like, but I don't think that I feel it as much because I am not actually smiling. I have started to write a diary . . . Writing it out helps a lot. Such and such has happened and I *feel* this. Writing allows me to express."

It seemed very likely that losing facial animation meant not only losing expression and communication with others but led to a reduced intensity and delineation of feeling within oneself. "The face talks of feelings. If you cannot show, then you have to express them somehow, and a diary would seem a good way. I can imagine that with one side moving that may help the other side know what is needed, but with both sides of the face gone, you may find it difficult to know exactly how to move it."[2]

"Yes, I know I feel that, so I keep practicing. I sit in front of a mirror, practicing for half an hour at a time."

A good friend of mine had had a similar bilateral facedrop in her early twenties and made a complete recovery. I told Oliver this, hoping for the same. I thanked him for allowing me to come. He in turn thanked me. In a new and unknown situation maybe I had been able to answer some of his questions. We agreed to meet a few months later.

There had been enormous improvement. He was able to move the upper half of his face well and though the mouth and lower face were still weak he could close his mouth to eat and drink, and was well enough to hold a cigarette between his lips. I asked if getting better had allowed him to look back on what it was like to be deprived of facial movement and all that entails, for few if any people had done this previously. His reply went far beyond what I had anticipated.

"Yes, I think so. I feel the whole condition has changed me enormously. Before, I was not at ease with myself and now I am. Just over the last few weeks I have reached a point when I am content with who I am. Because of my eyes there were weeks and months when I could not read or watch TV: that allowed self-contemplation. I think I was halfway there but now I have changed to a great extent. One of the things that helped me a lot was listening to extracts of Brian Keenan's book.[3] He was talking from within a cell and I felt trapped within my own cell myself. I could relate to what he went through.

"I felt like someone always wearing a mask, but not as you might expect. The facial problem was a bit like a mask, a mask of anonymity, partly because I was shy and uncertain of myself. But a mask can also act as a protective barrier—my face became such a mask for me and I was hiding behind it and getting more confidence.

"Then, knowing that people would be unsure of me because of my condition, it made me, enabled me, to be more forceful and less hesitant. I became more positive. I made more effort to communicate verbally and by gesture. I would wave my arms around like a Frenchman."

That such a huge loss of function had actually been beneficial was extraordinary. I paraphrased Wittgenstein, that the face is transparent and allows you see through it—to the person, to the soul.

"My soul, I think, was more in my voice. I noticed that on the telephone I had difficulty in controlling my own emotional state because I could not control my face—my face did tie in with this. You can be in a foul mood normally and speak on the phone as though happy. With the condition I could no longer do that. I could not lie."

Like Peter White, Oliver had come to reside in his voice. And with this there had been a stripping away of social games and pretense. Like John Hull's experience, it had become important to reduce ambiguity to a minimum. With both the voice and facial expression it was possible to give differing signals, say a deadpan expression with a laughing voice, and play one off the other. Without the two together then it seemed important to communicate one's true feelings clearly, and such social games were put aside.

"At Christmas, when my face was at its worst, I showed equal enthusiasm for each present. No one knew if I was pleased or not—a good thing, as long as I did not speak. I certainly found that in coming to terms with the face I was coming to terms with myself. It would not have been the same if I had broken a leg, because it was the face which forced me to come out of myself. And once I had got over something I became happier with myself because I had got over it. I find in the pub I get on better with the people there. I think now I am far more able to communicate with them.

"Once, when my illness was at its most severe, the postman came and gave me letters and I grinned, or did my best to. As he looked up he saw me. From then on he avoided my gaze. I knew he felt I had been insincere. It has allowed me a sense of compassion, for now I know what other people with a variety of problems have to face. One of the things I talked to people about was you interviewing me for your book. I didn't especially notice until then, but I was aware of them being aware of how they were reacting to me. It was probably a very good thing I said it, for it helped."

To have entered, even for a short time, the condition of Möbius must have been an almost unimaginable experience. Yet Oliver had not described purgatory, but refuge and sanctuary. He had been protected and supported, allowing contemplation of his enforced disconnection from display, and from the interrogation by others that facial expression allows. It had allowed an emotional and spiritual growth I had been unprepared for. Oliver Sacks, in his great epilogue to *Awakenings,* quotes Nietzsche:

Only great pain, the long, slow pain that takes its time . . . compels us to descend to our ultimate depths . . . I doubt if such pain makes us "better"; but I know it makes us more profound . . . one returns newborn, having shed one's skin . . . a hundred times subtler that one has ever been before.[4]

While the world saw only a mask, Oliver had explored ideas and feelings completely novel to him, and had returned more confident, compassionate, and mature. His temporary loss of facial animation had allowed him to reach an understanding of himself and of others.

Mrs. Doubtfire

Like Kafka's hero in *Metamorphosis,* when Brenda woke up she didn't know that anything was wrong. She made the tea and took some to her recently retired husband. It was only when she brought her own cup up to her mouth that she realized. She looked in the mirror: the left side of her face had fallen away, paralyzed. She ran to her husband, who said she had had a stroke. But she had seen her mother with a stroke and quickly checked her arms and legs. They were normal. No, she knew she had not had a stroke. She dressed and rushed to her doctor who said that she had Bell's palsy. He did not suggest any treatment. She returned home and stayed there, frightened by what had happened and too upset to show anyone outside her immediate family.

Like Gregor Samsa she soon discovered the obvious practical problems: she found it very difficult to eat and drink from a cup, so she used a child's beaker with a spout (a luxury when at home was to drink tea straight from a saucer).[5]

She went out little, if at all. Slowly, however, her face improved, and after four months she was practically back to normal, with a mild weakness that only a doctor or her family would recognize. Then, almost immediately, she developed a similar but less severe Bell's palsy on the right side. From here on, things became more complicated. For with the weakness on the right there began to be complications on the left. As the right side recovered a little she began to feel a tightness over her face. Her nose felt as though it was moving over to the right, and the contour of her face and its elasticity, which is so important for its function, was altering in ways she could not begin to understand.[6] Over the succeeding months she could no longer open her eyes and mouth easily. What had started off as a weakness was slowly becoming a tightened and fixed face, with her mouth a small unaltering oval. She could only put small morsels of food in it; cleaning her teeth was very difficult; kissing her husband, impossible.

At times she was very depressed, particularly about her eyes. Over one Christmas she was effectively blinded, not because she could not see with the eyes, but simply because the eyelids were shut by the overactivity of the facial muscles. Even before that she had run into severe difficulties. Because of the eyelids she couldn't see down, so she couldn't see the curb or the pavement to walk on. If this were not bad enough, she found that while she could not open her mouth fully, or smile, or make any facial expression, when she did attempt to shut her eyes her mouth grimaced upward involuntarily.[7]

We constantly seek to find meaning in random events. Brenda had remarried four years before the Bell's palsy and looked forward to a comfortable retirement with a new friend and companion. Her grown-up family from a previous marriage were all in favor of this and very supportive. Unfortunately, her husband Colin's family, were not. They were very hurtful and, worse, stopped coming around to see them. This was especially upsetting for Brenda because she had known Colin's son and daughter quite well before she met Colin. Colin was very upset by this and at times cried in front of her. She decided to keep all her feelings to herself and show nothing. All this had come to a head just before the Bell's palsy and she blamed the stress of this for the palsy. While there is no evidence to support such an idea, in her thoughts the bottling up of emotion merged with her face becoming devoid of facial expression altogether.

There was little that could be done about the mouth but she did see an ophthalmic surgeon. Minor operations reduced the size of her upper eyelids, and raised the eyebrows to lift the whole muscle and skin around the eye up and away from the pupil. The operations were not especially successful.

She made the most of it, however, and decided that she couldn't stay at home for the rest of her life. They invited friends around and explained the problem. It was not long before she realized that people treated her just as they always had. She was the same inside and her friends could see it.

Next, she went back to bingo, explaining with a laugh and a chuckle what the problem was and soon people got over their initial reservations. She went back to the village in which she had lived and worked for many years, either in the bakery or the greengrocery. Each time she met someone new she had to explain the problem, that her mandarin-like fixed face was only a mask and that she was back to her usual good-humored self. Being in her seventies, her oddly fixed face was not immediately apparent to people walking past her. Curiously though, it was apparent to children and, as children do, they used to come up and simply stare.[8] She didn't really know what to say: she'd have liked to explain what was wrong but knew she wouldn't be able to. So she had to let them stare or else walk away.

She had always loved to joke. Now, alas, she could make people laugh but could not produce a smile of her own. So she learned consciously to compensate for this. When she felt a smile come on she would laugh. The problem was that if she shut her eyes during this her mouth would grimace upward. So when she laughed she learned to move her hands over her face to avoid others' embarrassment and cover her own. At least laughter is loud. Without any ability to move her face she found it almost impossible to express sadness or empathy with friends who were going through bad times. She could overcome the mask that her face had become with humor, but the expression of less positive emotions drifted away from her. Despite the operations on her eyes the overactivity of the nerves persisted for years. She eventually met a surgeon who suggested injecting the muscles with a toxin, botulinum, which prevents muscular contraction. It seemed odd to have the nerves blocked when her original problem had been due to nerve damage but she was willing to try anything. She went along with her son and daughter. They were told that it would take three or four days. Her son remembers that after a day or so her eyes were wider. Not only could she see but, miraculously, there was also more of his mother to be seen on her face. By now she worried far less about what her face looked like, but did so want to see properly. The improvement caused by the drug lasted only a few months. For the last year or so she has been going back to have the injections and, thus far, they have proved reasonably successful. The surgeon has suggested that once she gets over this eye problem he might try injecting the mouth also.

Each time she goes to see him he asks if he might see her teeth in a smile. She swears that one day she's going to put her hand in her mouth and whip out her false teeth to show him. But she lives in hope that he will be so successful with the injections that one day her smile will return. If not, then she knows, and those around her know, that her natural resilience will carry her through. Only she knows, however, the alterations in her emotional life which her loss of facial movement has imposed. Unlike in Kafka's tale, Brenda's problem has not gone away. She has overcome it, as best she can, by transferring her self to her voice and gestures, and by a gloriously stubborn and bloody refusal to accept less of a life.

I nicknamed Brenda "Mrs. Doubtfire" because she was a little like the character Robin Williams played in the eponymous film. He had on so much facial makeup that he could no longer move his face. Both he and Brenda compensated for their lack of facial expression by increasing the animation of their speech and gestures.

Coming Alive—The Video

Oliver and Brenda suffered sudden, calamitous facial paralysis with differing responses. But for most people loss of facial animation occurs so slowly that, astonishingly, it may not be recognized.

Iona Lister is a speech therapist trained to assist patients in overcoming speech and language disorders. She works with patients with a range of conditions, from stroke to motor neuron disease. More recently, kindled by a single meeting, her interests have expanded to encompass another aspect of communication.

"I was working with a lady with Parkinson's disease. Chatting with her, I must confess, was stodgy and heavy going—just like the disease. Lastly, toward the end of the session, she mentioned that she had been very interested in art and she described some of the pictures she painted. She mentioned that she used to be involved in belly-dancing! Once I had left her I realized how surprised I was that she had such an interesting set of hobbies—as though in my mind I had decided that she was a rather dull, colorless person with no interests and with nothing attractive about her at all. I then realized why my impressions had been formed and was so amazed and ashamed, because here I was behaving just as I had been upbraiding the general public for behaving. I was judging her by her inability to be animated facially, and I should have known better.[9]

"I went onto a case conference about this lady and all my colleagues described her as being drab and uninteresting. The physical therapist thought she would not need to go up and down steps because she would not have much of a social life. Her whole persona, which had been projected through a lack of facial animation (for her speech was normal, not even monotonous as some people with Parkinson's become), had led to various assumptions about her lifestyle. It was only because I had listened that I learned about the richness of her life and then realized, not without some shame, how and why I had judged her."

I asked if her patient had been aware of people's perceptions of her and if she perceived herself as others did.

"She was unaware of the way she was perceived. I managed to introduce it in what I hoped was a sensitive manner and she was interested in my observations. She came back a couple of weeks later saying that she had decided it was a problem. We decided to work on her facial expression, consciously, together."

After that Iona found herself more and more interested in the problems of lack of facial animation that some people with Parkinson's experience. She became involved with the local Parkinson's Disease Society, which met once a month for a social gathering, and immediately discerned the social dynamics of the meeting.

"I didn't set out to observe this, but it came to me with a thundering clarity, and I saw the same on many subsequent occasions. It was that if, in the group of forty attenders and people with Parkinson's, there might be five with facial problems, and people tended not to gravitate toward those. Not only that, but often their partner rather than them would be asked how they were. People would ask these facially impoverished people questions that demanded yes or no answers rather than more expansive ones, so avoiding an engaged conversation."

Iona decided that, after a certain amount of this perception of being boring and unsocial, these people imperceptibly may have become asocial and withdrawn. A self-fulfilling hypothesis, like the "beauty is good" one, perhaps.

"There was a definite movement away from these people at the meetings. Perhaps people did not get any feedback from the patients and so did not feel engaged and encouraged. The other thing was that the husbands and wives of these patients appeared to be compensating, even overcompensating. They were very chatty and even overpowering. The message seemed to be to the Parkinson's patient, 'You just sit there and have a good time, I can do the talking for a bit and perhaps forget about your needs for a while.'"

I wondered with this if the patient's self-esteem was lowered with impoverishment of expression and if then an element almost of condescension, however unconsciously, entered into their relationships.

"A face which does not fit into the socially acceptable says, 'Don't come here, you will not receive gratification.' In a film I saw recently about a young child with a facial disfigurement, the child has good compensating techniques to engage you and make her attractive. It is rarely like that in real life, unfortunately. In the movies they all seem to have superhuman skills and their disability has not damaged their confidence. What about those who are not specially talented?"

This was an important point. It is certainly the case that, outside Hollywood, people with facial problems lose confidence so that their abilities to overcome the problem are lessened. What may seem a small facial problem to us may be a source of almost insuperable misery to them, and they may not learn to cope on their own.

"They have social isolation on two levels. One, a static unattractiveness, in that they are just sitting there, and the human face, when not putting on quirky unusual expressions as it does when there are people around, tends to become set and to look rather petulant and glum. That is what people actually see in a resting face in these patients. Then, when the face does start to move, it is elaborating all sorts of things about what we are saying. For example, as I sit here talking you are reading my movements. That adds to the attractiveness. The subtlety of communication is complemented by the face: wrong clues can actually alter meaning. If you say, 'Nice to see you,' with no facial movement or with the wrong movement, it can actually appear sarcastic or whatever.

"These patients are patronized, isolated, and lose acknowledgment of themselves. I showed my film to a group of parkinsonian people and at the end of it one man said, 'How awful, I'm glad I'm not like that." I nearly left my chair because if anyone had facial immobility, it was him. I wondered, should I confront him or not? I had a fairly close relationship with his partner and I asked her the best way to bring it up. It was brought up and he went through the program. It only had a limited effect because he did it on sufferance. His wife was nagging and he did not want to disappoint me, so he just went through the motions."

"Perhaps with a chronic progressive neurological disease, he knew he wasn't going to break out, so he may have retreated from it. In pointing it out were you showing him what he was trying to turn away from, toward a more intact world as best he could find within himself?"

"What I was trying to show was that he had an option. Just by participating and with the will to govern what normally takes care of itself, facial expression, he could enrich his life despite the disease."

I asked what she had done to improve facial expressiveness in these patients.

"I went to various books and articles to look up what was being done. There is not very much. An article on communication devoted much space to voice, intonation, posture, all the usual things, with little on facial expression. Then it was all so dry and boring. 'Ask the patient to practice smiling and grimacing,' and I thought that if you tell them to do that, they won't do it because it does not mean anything. So I decided to devise a program which would involve them appreciating others' facial expressions. At the beginning I ask people to turn off the sound of the TV while watching a soap and get them to understand various emotions. Newsreaders are good at adding color to reading, and we asked them to do this too."

More important, perhaps, she also found time to research, write, and direct a video showing people some of the things they can do to recover facial expression.[10]

The film begins with four people enjoying a game of cards around a table, drinking wine and laughing. But as the camera pans around the table you realize that one of the four is not laughing, and that she has the rather severe and impassive rigidity of the face sometimes seen in people with Parkinson's. Whereas the others show their enjoyment and emotion via their animated and constantly moving faces, this woman cannot. It is explained that the woman can smile or frown if she thinks about it, but that in general conversation it does not usually happen on its own. As a consequence she is left out, and this can happen without anyone being aware of it. The person is simply considered rather dull and boring, without anyone asking why.

"Having demonstrated an appreciation of the importance of facial expression in a client we then go on to some stimulation and tapping and brushing of the face. It just makes them feel tingly and makes them focus on the face. I just tell them it makes the face come alive. There are so few licenses to touch in society that it allows them or their carers to do this. They love the icing and tapping. It is also important to establish rapport."

The video suggests they set aside a time to themselves and go to a quiet place initially once a day but then, after a few weeks, less frequently. First they are asked to relax—"It is your time to enjoy yourself." They go through a series of tapping over the face with two fingers, then ice wrapped in gauze is stroked over the face. Then they are asked to move the face and hold it in a variety of expressions, whistling, smiling, frowning, and yawning. These are reinforced by holding the eyebrows up with the fingers and closing the eyes against resistance, or by placing the fingers in the mouth and trying to shut the lips on them. They are asked to try to feel what they are doing and feel the muscles tighten.

"I can imagine that if the face has not moved expressively for some time, then one might forget the right expression and movement, and forget how to achieve this. They may need to look because they have lost confidence in their ability to feel inside."

"I sometimes wonder if people with a growing disability, especially Parkinson's, as their condition is deteriorating, lose that inner knowledge, or respect for, or interest in, or care for their own bodies."

I suggested that people with chronic problems might live within themselves more, and withdraw from their face and from the world, thinking of James trying to live entirely within his head. The face is a privileged place for communication with both the world and with oneself. Iona replied,

"I had a car when it was new, and I was always cleaning it and looking at it from all angles. I was proud of it and invested it with a personality. Now it is six years old, and over the years the dog has clawed the back, people have dented it, and one headlight is bashed in. It is looking pretty tatty and now it is just an object—a thing. I don't give it a name; it is purely functional. I have disinvested it and neglected it. Do people do that with their own bodies?"

"So by using their face maybe you are giving them a chance to reinvest."

"There is something awful about having a crappy car and lavishing care on it and being proud of it. Perhaps a deteriorating body makes you neglect it to keep your self-respect. In the exercises, I don't use the word 'exercise.' If you say, "Go away and do your exercise once a day,' then they will not do it. Instead, I say that this is your time to treat yourself, to pamper yourself, *your* treat for *you*. Then they do the exercises, which help, but they are also investing time in themselves, and respecting their body, connecting with it. After the exercises I ask them to imagine certain statements and react to them, for example, 'Look at that big spider,' or 'I have just reversed my car into yours,' and then they try to generalize into conversations. I will ask, 'What have you been doing today?' Open questions to get them responding both in words and facially."

The video suggests that they use news broadcasts and imagine the reader is in the room with them so they have to react to the news with facial expressions. In this way they can rehearse before using the regained skills in natural conversation. It is suggested that they may have to think about their faces for a while, then soon the animation will take care of itself and occur once more without thought.

"You never say, 'Look happy,' rather you give them appropriate, funny situations?"

"That's right, because it is their response. I am not telling them how to feel in a given situation but just to respond. If they want to laugh, then that's part of their personality and OK. Then progressively we encourage them to move into society. It does involve the cooperation of the partner for support and help. People have to be motivated. It is their prerogative to decide one way or the other. If they contemplate the face dangling a little in front of them they may see the entirety of their problem. It tends to work for those for whom communication has been very important for most of their lives, like teachers—the more outgoing, those who have been more socially skilled.

"The loss of facial animation does not engage sympathy from others like a broken leg may. Loss of facial animation is completely different; the disease may actually not engage sympathy at all. Quite the reverse."

"You are saying 'I am dull and boring.' And it may be worse because with Parkinson's the change is interpreted as a loss of interest."[11]

Despite my protestations Iona had bought me lunch as we chatted through the afternoon. As we walked through north Oxford to our cars I asked if she could send me the addresses of some patients who had used the video. A little while later she gave me a few names, none of whom she knew, for she did not want their relationship with her to cloud their honesty about her program.

Grumpy

Edward, who has Parkinson's disease, and his wife Helen live in a small town in the Thames Valley. They have recently moved to a new house within walking distance of the center. Though we had spoken over the phone I had no idea how severe Edward's Parkinson's was. I was met by a couple in their mid-seventies, a little wary, as well they might be, but full of life. Edward showed the difficulties in walking and voluntary movement typical of the disease, and the mild, smooth involuntary movements of the head seen sometimes as a side effect of medication. However, one would have passed him in the street without remarking on his face.

Helen told me that it had started over ten years ago. They had been driving in the car listening to the radio. That morning a doctor was discussing Parkinson's disease and mentioned that in some cases the facial expression becomes more rigid, and the person appears dull and grumpy. She looked across at her husband, a man who had been full of good humor and fun, and thought that he had it. However, the thought passed; she did not mention it to Edward then (and still had not until I had talked with them). They were newly retired and as one gets older, she reasoned, one's face does become less animated.

Two years went by. One of Edward's many hobbies had been photography and he had built up a large library which he used to give talks to local groups.

"I used to do a lot of talks on churches, bridges, and canals from a layman's point of view. I went to a local meeting two miles away and gave a talk. I came home and did not know how I had got home, nor did I remember how I had given the talk."

He had never had any problems with his memory before and so the next day went along to his doctor who arranged for him to see a neurologist, whose interest was in amnesia. After the usual brain scans and psychological reports the neurologist was able to reassure Edward that the amnesia was not going to happen again. The bad news, however, was that he had Parkinson's disease, a complete shock, for Edward himself had not noticed any symptoms.

For the next five years he continued on a small amount of medication. Helen remembers little difference in Edward's use of the face during this time. Though hardly aware that he was more disinterested and poorer company, she did find herself answering more for him, partly to speed up matters and partly to cover Edward's dullness. Edward was never aware of this, and she never once mentioned to Edward that his face made him look miserable. Then a new doctor suggested a visit to a physiotherapist and to a speech therapist who was interested in Parkinson's.

"I have lived all my life by my mouth, being a teacher and doing amateur drama, and I had, by this time, found myself less able to join in conversations. I had never had that before and I had no idea why. Maybe it was psychological or mental, a mental block to prevent me having opinions to voice. I still did not know my face was affected at all. I would have disagreed if anyone had said that I was in that situation.

"The speech therapist did not think she could do anything from the articulatory point of view, but she knew Iona Lister and gave me the booklet and the video. It was very dramatic, I immediately recognized myself as being like the woman in the video. I had not realized that I had facial symptoms, but then I immediately understood that the face could have explained some of the problems.

"We did the icing, the tapping and stroking together. I would do the exercises in front of a mirror. I had always thought that with the teaching and acting that I was quite mobile with the face, but quickly realized this was no longer the case. By doing the exercises I freed up my face and then it moved again automatically. I did not seem to move it consciously."

The process of giving the face exercises seemed sufficient to get it moving once again, and these movements slowly became subconscious, to some extent at least.

"When I went back to talking with people I noticed that I was moving my face more. Since the exercises I have been a bit more confident. I am more aware of where my face is than before."

"But normally we are not aware of what our face is doing."

"That is right, it just comes with the words. I was never aware that I looked a little vacant. I realize now that that is why people were not involving me in conversation."

On the one hand, the problem seemed to have been that he did not have much to say, but also on the other that, because of the face immobility, people simply did not involve and engage him. The face was essential for conversation and for the figure of eight with others. Not only did he have little to say but there was no one to listen. Even Helen would talk to him and get no reaction and so think that he was not interested, so they would talk less and less.

"I thought I was bothering him. Since the therapy it has been much better. The monotony of the voice is far better. When he retired he wanted to do talking books for the blind, but the voice was so monotonous that they did not accept him. He has come alive again since the facial exercises, I have to remind him of that every so often. He is a jolly fellow, but when he looks miserable all the time, it *is* gloomy. After the video I was surprised at the difference it made. In the church choir he would not open his mouth to sing. Now he can, and the sound now comes out far better. It has helped enormously in conversations with the family. On the phone people have said how much better Edward performs and how much more lively he sounds."

But the video had been only about facial movement, I said. Helen explained that she had noticed how, when talking on the phone, the face moves as though you are conversing face to face with someone. So that if the face could be reanimated then the voice followed. It did not end there, however.

Reanimation of his face had led to a general return of interest and enthusiasm for everything. Maybe that was telling us something about the importance of the face for emotional experience. Perhaps it was too simple to think of different channels of expression: body language, speech, and face. Edward's experience suggests that they are linked and interdependent. They were so at home and delightful to be with that it was hard to discuss the seven years or so when the disease had either been undiagnosed, or diagnosed and treated with no thought for the face. At one stage they had filled out social work forms, about mobility, about walking distance, about stairs, but never about the face. Yet in Edward's case it was the face that seemed, in retrospect, to hold a key to the emotional and social impoverishment which Parkinson's imposed.

Oliver and Brenda had been very aware of their loss of facial animation. For one it was a refuge from social interaction and inquisition, for the other a source of isolation and frustration. One had recovered and returned to his world infinitely richer; the other through force of personality had overcome it despite little functional improvement. In contrast, in Parkinson's disease the loss was unseen, though its consequences were not. Wittgenstein wrote, "We do not see facial contortions and make the inference that he is feeling joy . . . We describe a face immediately as sad, radiant, bored . . . "

In some people with Parkinson's the face is transparent and we go straight through it to consider the person dull and boring, with no realization that our perceptions originate from a facial problem. Until, that is, someone like Iona comes along. And her experience suggests that the face is not an isolated part of our approach to, and communication with, the world, but is essential both for the engagement and relatedness which underpins our social existence, and for emotional self-expression too. From the way in which Oliver found that he could not lie with the voice when his face was "inanimate," and from Edward's reanimation of voice and body language when he was able to move his face more, it is probably simplistic to think of these differing areas for emotional communication as being separate. Maybe the face, expressing emotion to others and to self, is first among equals in this. The face, after all, is the first place for emotional communication in babies.

Now imagine being like this from birth. Perhaps then it becomes apparent why James used body language and even speech so little, and why he tried to live "in his head." For never having known facial animation, he was perhaps less embodied in other channels of expression and communication as well. His narrative certainly suggested a primacy for facial expression for emotional experience and communication.

.

Changing Faces

11

Autism is a most private world, perhaps the most private of existences, a world so private that it has been glimpsed only by way of fragmented autobiographical accounts and can hardly be shared, even between fellow autistic persons. In Parkinson's disease emotionless faces are also private, but in the sense that they are seen straight through, and not recognized for what they are.

In contrast, the most public of all faces is a disfigured one. A disfigured face is always on display, so that often people come up to the disfigured, curiosity overcoming respect. Disfigurement may come to define a person's whole existence and persona. It was to this group that I turned finally, not to categorize or consider their faces, but to see how they came to terms with them and how they asserted their independence and individuality.

Seven Years of Trial and Error

They never got to go hill walking in Wales. Driving one night to a favorite haunt, James Partridge's Land Rover toppled over at a bend in the road. His friends struggled out fast, but James, though saved from being knocked unconscious by his seat belt, was caught by some wreckage. As he was lying flat on his seat the fire started. By the time he had got out he had been burned severely over his body, hands, and face. A couple passing by saved him, the woman's fur coat keeping him warm for the vital few minutes before he was admitted to the hospital.

Shocked and severely burned, he was rushed to intensive care. After the first period of resuscitation he was moved to a surgical ward for the early skin grafts and then more measured reconstructive surgery. After months of this he was discharged and then, at last, took up his course at Oxford, going back for further plastic surgery on vacations. Left with a scarred hand and a beautiful patchwork face, he became a health economist, then a farmer and part-time teacher in the Channel Islands.

Married by now and with a family, he had returned to the able world, and could have consigned his burns to the past, an increasingly forgotten nightmare. Or he could have written an inspiring account of his experiences. His recovery was not through miracles of plastic surgery making him "normal" again (though the surgery was miraculous, that much was beyond them), but by confronting his disfigurement, by embracing it, and by inviting others to see through it and finally to realize that it was irrelevant.

He did not write that book. Instead he wrote a book—a wonderful book—in simple and accessible prose about his experiences, not with him as hero or even as him as central figure, but a classic user's guide and textbook for all those with facial disfigurement.[1] He told of the feelings and practical difficulties experienced in recovering from a facial burn, and of a host of other difficulties someone with a changed face has to meet. For instance, immediately after the injury he was put in a germ-free ward to prevent infection. He saw only nurses and doctors gowned and masked. He soon discovered that the good nurses seemed to accentuate their eye movements and body language instinctively, to compensate for the loss of communication resulting from their masks. He began to realize very soon that his world had changed in unexpected ways.

He describes in his book when and how to look at your face for the first time after a burn. He found that his visitors often needed to be shown how to talk to him and be put at their ease. He soon realized that people do not know how to react to facial disfigurement. He, as the disfigured person, was the expert at helping those around him. He discusses how to cope with the inevitable staring when returning to the world outside. The book is written in such open, dispassionate prose that one is hardly aware of the cost of this knowledge, either in terms of the disfigurement, or of the personal misery over many years, which lay behind the learning. Only once or twice does he mention this past, when reflecting on the fact that each day he meets new people and has to display his face anew.

In Britain the book was such a great success that he was invited to appear on a TV talk show. A fellow guest was a psychologist, Nicola Rumsey, who had written her doctoral dissertation on disfigurement. James and Nicola started chatting afterwards and began to realize that though they had been approaching the experience of facial disfigurement from opposite poles, they had come to startlingly similar conclusions: that there was a gap in health care after plastic surgery had done its best. What happened to disfigured people then? They were not being helped to cope with their new faces and not being shown how to cope in the company of others. Nicola's research and James's practical experience had convinced them both that such people needed help in returning to a full life in society.

Over the next few weeks and months they met and talked about what needed to be done. They decided to set up a charity called, like the book, "Changing Faces." They needed money, buildings, staff, and publicity. James had some friends and started lobbying and cajoling the rich and influential. He became figurehead and publicist, fundraiser and organizer. A place was found in London and start-up funds were raised. At some risk he gave up his job and threw himself into the project full-time. As soon as funds and facilities were sufficient, they advertised for clients. Their approach was to view disfigurement as being initially a sort of bereavement, followed by a tremendous, almost overpowering, sense of inadequacy and isolation. Their aim was somehow to enable disfigured persons to recover their feelings of self-worth, building on their talents, and acquiring the confidence to go out into the world and manage the way in which other people responded to them.

People with facial disability often became passive and retiring, only reacting to other people, never initiating and controlling conversations or decisions. They had to be given help to actually manage their social relationships in their own way and to their own advantage. Through disabled grapevines and appearances on radio and television they attracted clients and invited them to a two-day workshop. At the workshops they emphasized social skills and social interaction: If you obtain positive responses from those you meet, then your sense of self-respect and self-worth will increase. They taught that social relationships work on feedback, both positive and negative.

They soon realized that the first thing was to ask clients to do something that most found extraordinarily difficult: to look one another straight in the face and describe their problems. They sought a shared experience of disability and loss. They asked people to focus on their bad experiences, to talk about them in front of complete strangers, in a new place far from home. There was a collective sense of horror, a shared reliving of their worst times. By confronting and making explicit the worst experiences, all were able to realize the magnitude of what was required. The people who came to their workshops had all sorts of problems, from burns or the effects of cancer operations, to those whose imperfections appeared to be of mild severity but which were causing profound problems. To their initial surprise, James and Nicola found no simple relation between the physical and the perceived disfigurement.

The depth of the problem was illustrated by one man who said, "I avoid public transport, I avoid going to parties, I avoid going anywhere where I don't know people. I avoid going anywhere I will be stared at, I cannot cope, I just turn my face away. I find myself so unattractive that I feel I should not be mixing with others. I feel as if I am letting the side down. I get nervous, and that makes the other person nervous. I give out bad vibes."

In planning the workshops James and Nicola were aware of how vulnerable people would be. They knew that many people would have spent years walling up the problem, and that they needed to see the enemy before they could begin to take it on. Munch's famous painting *The Scream* is powerful in part because the cause of the anxiety is not shown. People needed to see the cause before they could find ways around it.

The vulnerability, though precarious and vertiginous, was also necessary for the next stage. Each person had to realize and understand that he or she was not unique. The person had to realize that he or she needed the one thing that was so difficult, not only to get by, but to be healed. To regain social currency and recover self-esteem it was necessary to reach out to others. James and Nicola suggested ways in which this might be done, which many of those with facial problems could not conceive of themselves as being able to do. One client suggested that the problems were so enormous that he did not believe any strategy to manage social relationships was possible.

They discussed how not all groups of people are the same. Loved ones, family, and immediate friends, those who have known one from the beginning may be relied on. Nurses and professionals, who are trained to react in certain ways and to be aware of certain problems, may be another group not too difficult to approach. But strangers may react in a different and distressing way. Clients had to be made aware of these differences in order to cope.

It would be wonderful if the rest of the world knew something of facial disfigurement. Then facially disfigured people might not have to do anything. Some might think that's good, but would it really be? For there is an element of pity in this, and anyway no one can wait long enough for the world to come round to this way of thinking. They had to realize that the world probably never will be able to cope with facial disfigurement—there is something that makes many people turn away from various forms of physical and mental disability.

At the workshops clients were made to realize that they have to take the initiative and make people respond to them. They stressed that disfigured people have to manage their own lives and manage meetings with others not in a milieu of pity but as people, just like anyone else. James and Nicola used acronyms like *reach out*—Reassurance, Energy, Assertiveness, Courage, Humor, Otherness, Understanding, and Tolerance—and worked through these ideas discussing new skills as they went.

Disfigured people needed reassurance that they are not in an "I can't do anything" situation. If they do not expect people to make eye contact with them, they can *make* them do it. They also needed to reassure others. If people with facial disabilities don't feel they can look someone in the eye the end of their nose may do (it is difficult for someone to realize that the gaze is actually directed at the nose). If they can't move the skin around the eyes, for whatever reason, they can use the forehead or the mouth. If they don't feel they can move their face, they are taught to use the body and arms, or the voice. Use what is left, but use it.

The clients received reassurance from the group and, more important, were taught to give it to those they meet, for the general public are awkward when faced with a disfigured person. Someone with a facial disability needs to reassure people that he or she is normal and available for normal conversation and interaction. Shaking hands can, for instance, put people at ease and James taught how to do even this simple thing, which requires confidence and timing.

All people with disabilities, of whatever sort, have to try harder to function socially, and this requires energy. They have to learn that they will live at a higher energy state, whether it be in their posture or in their desire to reach out to people. Life does become more difficult in terms of what one has to put into it, but it can also become more rewarding. People with facial disability have to be aware that people may stare at them and be sarcastic. They don't have to be passive recipients; they need to be able to reach the right level of self-projection to cope with such comments or to prevent them occurring in the first place, something that tone of voice and general aspect helps with.

The very act of coming to a Changing Faces workshop may have required an enormous amount of courage. The aim of these little group sessions is to give people a resilience to go out into the world and overcome their natural inclination to hide. James and Nicola aim to give courage, to encourage, and this is done most effectively through sharing. They encourage their clients to encourage those they meet to treat them as they would anyone else.

People may be laughed with, and laughed at, and they need to be able to enter into this, for if people sense you can't see the funny side of something they may turn away.

People with a facial disability can be very self-conscious. They may go to an interview or other social situation terrified, so terrified that they are not aware of other people, for that awareness comes through watching, something they may shy away from. They need to become attuned to the ways other people approach them and their disability so that they can manipulate it. They often do not know how to do this but there are some simple ways.

Open-ended questions like, "What work do you do?" or "What do you do?" which require a sentence or two in answering, encourage people to talk about themselves and keep the conversation flowing. To be conscious of others reduces self-consciousness. It works both ways: the newly met person, when talking about himself or herself, won't be thinking about the person with the disability. They, in turn, may ask the disabled person about himself or herself and the disability will fade away.

Some workshops, in fact, are just about conversational skills: how to begin and end a conversation and how to remove the distraction of the disfigurement. In these and many other exercises the aim is to establish the two-way flow that conversation requires, thus building a relationship.

People with facial disability need a range of behaviors, a repertoire of skills at different times, and an armamentarium to deal with abuse. They must deal with people at different levels of intimacy, and have ways of being in situations ranging from dances to funerals. Initially they may feel like actors and consider that what they're doing has a level of falsity, but they are reassured that skills can be developed through consciousness to become unconscious (in the jargon, from unconscious incompetence through conscious incompetence, to conscious competence to unconscious competence, the "cycle of learning").

Clients are made to realize that, though they may become expert at some social situations, there will always be new situations to cope with—the first time on a beach, the first time in a pub, the first time back at work, the first time with new people, the first time seeing one's uncle after a number of years. Disfigurement is a lifetime challenge.

In his book James does not emphasize it, but it is clear how long and difficult a passage it was for him to accept and them live with his own changed face. (In his own words, "seven years of trial and error.") It is only when the owner of the face accepts his or her disfigurement that he or she is ready to help others to do so. The catch is that true acceptance, for the owner, is not a matter of being at one with the changed face at home or with friends, but of being able to go out into the world. The courage to expose oneself, actively and vulnerably, must be part of the process. We live not "in our own heads" but exist, and are made whole, in the reflective mirror of others.

I was keen to meet someone who had been on the receiving end at a series of workshops. James wrote to a few people, and that is how I came one evening to be talking with Jenny.

Seeing the Enemy

Jenny had herpes zoster (shingles) when she was nine years old, which affected the upper two thirds of her face. An unsightly scar formed and her nose became rather large and bulbous. It was red and would sweat at odd and very embarrassing times. She had several operations with varying degrees of success. Though initially not bothered, her embarrassment and awkwardness worsened as she got older. By the age of twelve she was using camouflage makeup continually and during her teens she had several operations to reduce the size and curvature of her nose. They were not a great success. By sixteen she was desperate, bullied at school, and nicknamed "Concorde." Her reaction was to shy away: "I would not retort or fight. This was characteristic of the whole. I tried to deny that it was there. I used to stop at home. It changed my life, for before the herpes I was quite outgoing and confident. I was no longer interested in relationships."

Her last operation was at age twenty-three. She had gone to the doctor and asked if there was anything else that could be done, a courageous thing to do, for asking for a change in one's face is not like asking for antibiotics. A skin graft across the nose gave an excellent cosmetic result. But by then her social difficulties were so much a part of her that she hardly connected them with her face—they *were* her, part of her (just as James Brown blamed himself and not the Möbius syndrome).

"Even going through that did not make me think consciously that there was anything different about me. I still was very shy and hung up, and did not connect it with the face and my facial disfigurement. Even after the surgery I still thought people were noticing it, and it was almost worse than having, say, a big black spot, because I was never sure if people stared, or if it was my imagination. Camouflage may have made me look normal but it was not any different on the inside."

Then one evening, two years later, she heard a program on the radio in which the new charity Changing Faces was discussed. She was aware that at some level she felt depressed, but "I had never attributed it to anything in particular, least of all imagined that it could have something to do with my looks."

One person on the program made a comment about low self-esteem—a revelation to Jenny, who realized she felt the same. She wrote off and then attended a workshop, sixteen years after her problem had originated. By this time, shy, withdrawn, and hardly knowing if the problem was her or her face, hardly ever looking at her face or at herself, she existed in a world of diminished self-worth, a world of jeopardy.

"At the workshop people expressed their experience and their anger. I began to think perhaps there is something of that in me too. After the highs of university, and an M.A. degree, I had a job, but I was frightened to go out. The language used at the workshop was very strong. They felt isolated, worthless, inadequate. One feels so terrible in oneself. Then other people can read those messages, and they send them back. To actually reach out to someone else when you have a facial disfigurement is enormously difficult. On the first visit no one looked at each other."

James Partridge had begun by making people extraordinarily vulnerable, more vulnerable perhaps than they had been for years, as vulnerable as they had been at the time of their injury. Many had been disfigured for years and existed by blotting out their problems as best they could. Changing Faces was breaking through this, and started without giving anything back.

"We also had to sit around and draw some pictures: what was important in our lives, where we saw ourselves right now. I drew my parents and the three dogs, and me away from them. No one else was there. It was extraordinarily depressing—the emotions that people were feeling and expressing made it very heavy. We would break for coffee and we all sat drinking with no talk and no looking at each other."

As I listened, Jenny held her hand over the left side of her face, midway between holding back her long hair from her face and scratching the side of her nose. In fact, it was to cover what I saw as a small scar on the bridge of her nose, and which did not appear to detract from her beauty.

"We did a fair amount on why you feel so bad about the face. A couple of people actually said that they had tried to commit suicide."

Then they tried to put it together again. They role-played.

"Someone said that they found it difficult on the train, so we played at this. We had to make eye contact with strangers. I could do it, but I was aware that I was very aggressive, staring, I just couldn't look with the right weight. Eye contact is so important and yet so difficult. One lady found it difficult on a bus. What does she do, get out a paper or look out the window?"

Even occasions that are public but not social were difficult.

"We were led through making eye contact and shown how to concentrate on body language, and empowerment, and the thing of you getting something back from people. We looked at how people felt about their face and what it was that made them feel like that. To actually make people realize that there was something tangible there, that if you could not alter it, then you could change how you feel about it and the way others feel about it. We plummeted the depths of what we felt and then saw what could be done. You have to name the enemy. It was the first time I started to admit the problem."

I suggested that to turn one's back on one's face must be to deny a very deep part of oneself.

"Yes, you have to see the enemy. You have to reveal the depths of the way you are feeling. In the past people may have had a problem but got by ignoring it, or put up with it."

"Perhaps facial problems become buried, or are so obvious that they are hardly seen. Perhaps people become dislocated from the cause of their feelings of inadequacy?"

"Yes, I think that is true. Certainly in my experience a lot of the time I was low it was not only the face—the face was almost forgotten. A lot of others were saying that."

Making contact with other people helped, certainly when people gave their reasons for feeling as they did, acknowledging the pain. It was cathartic to finally unburden and let go. But there was still resistance. She came out of the second day of the workshop and walked to the subway with someone, wanting to know, "Was I all right in the talk?" Whatever people had said at the session she had not really believed them. She realized that the workshop couldn't help because she wouldn't let it. Going back next day she let go more.

"At the end I felt liberated. The floodgates had been opened, I began to realize just how bad I felt about myself, and that perhaps it *could* be something to do with my face, that it explained many of my feelings. It was unanimous that we would go away feeling inspired and better for the two days, but everyone also felt a great sense of sadness. Then, as I started thinking, I felt stripped of everything and I did not know where to start to pick up the pieces."

The course was over a Thursday and Friday. Clients were encouraged to be honest with themselves, and to express their feelings and describe—perhaps for the first time—how their experience of facial disfigurement had affected their lives. Jenny had learned more about the making of eye contact, about her dark clothes, and the hand over the bridge of her nose. Yet over the weekend she felt very fragile and down, and this carried on for some time after. What could she do now? The two days were obviously not enough, so she wrote again to Changing Faces. James invited her to see him and that started a series of fifteen to twenty one-on-one meetings over the next few months. They helped her become aware of the issues.

"Previously I had been going through the motions. The meetings helped me to explore the issues in my own way in my own time. I was helped to gain self-esteem, partly by example, for if he could do it, then so could I. But that was not all. Much of it was exploring issues raised by myself, giving it all time to settle. At times I had wanted the problem to be big. If friends had said my scar was hardly noticeable I felt awful. Yet if they said it was a huge blemish, then that would have been terrible too. I was trying to lead them on to say the right thing, trying to trap them to tell me what I wanted."

She also went to further workshops on communication skills. Some were more useful than others, but she kept going since by now there was no way out, nowhere else to go.

Some of the others went for support, but Jenny did not want that; she did not want to be close only to people with problems. A problem for any support group is to give both mutual support and community, and yet also encourage people to let go and go out into the world.

"There's nothing that can be done to make it easier except to have an understanding ear. I can see that now, in retrospect. At the time I felt I needed all the support there was. Going through it was excruciating. There were times, many times, when I wished that I had never switched on the radio that day, and I had never heard of Changing Faces. It had exposed the wound. At the time I felt it was worsening it. If I tried to explain to people why . . . I half thought I was going mad. My disquiet about going was in part because it brought it out, anger, mourning, and so forth. I had denied it. If I am completely honest I felt this way about the exercise until recently. It took nearly two years. That was a period of mourning. It was leaving the mourning behind which coincided with me developing other ways of coping and going into the world."

In retrospect she feels that in the six months after the first workshop that she may have had a nervous breakdown, such were her feelings of pain and anxiety. Confusion, despair, and complete uncertainty—around and around she thought, were her feelings anything to do with the scarring on her face or not?

"Thankfully that is now in the past, though even now there are situations when I wonder if people stare. This new house has something wrong, and I have to go to the site office; that is still an ordeal. I do not find it easy to approach new people. I still get tongue-tied, and find myself saying, Hold on, slow down. I accept the way I look, and feel that I have more control over my feelings. Changing Faces has had a beneficial effect on my life, though at the time the experience was far from pleasurable."

"What would have happened had you not switched the radio on?"

"I think I would have carried on in my own withdrawn world. I don't think as many people would be in my life as there are now. I have learned about other people at work and I can empathize with them. I can see how I was, and how they are. I now have more of an insight into people. OK, my problem is visible, but I can see into others better, whether they have visible, physical problems or not."

For in the end Changing Faces is not only about disfigurement: its message, that it is possible to think about social skills and become empowered, is applicable to all. In those with facial problems speech and gesture become more important. In the spinally injured the face may be the main area of affective communication. Jenny describes her time with the charity as being among the hardest of her life, but after two years of mourning and searching and trying to build self-confidence she is now able to go out into the world. Now, perhaps for the first time, she can look at others, look into their faces, and not just see herself reflected, confident of reading the theory of mind of those around her. She can be aware enough to feel their weaknesses and begin to realize that most of us, the able bodied, have problems too. She has gone from hardly daring to feel, to feeling for others.

Changing Faces has been established as a charity for about three and a half years, and has seen approximately 1200 adults and 250 children. To continue the work it needs to become incorporated into the health system. James and Nicola's idea was that, just as the spinally injured have a period in a specialist unit, so those coping and coming to terms with facial problems should also. For the last year or so they have been soliciting funds and seeking facilities to set up a unit in a hospital. As a result of their hard work, and James's endless charm and good spirits, they opened the first disfigurement support unit, "Outlook," in the United Kingdom, in Bristol, early in 1995. They will need to satisfy the accountants and the managers of its usefulness. Confidence and self-esteem are difficult to measure, but Nicola has a battery of psychological tests at hand: anxiety and depression scales, avoidance and distress scales, questionnaires on motivation, coping skills. They are now underway with various grants for a couple of years. After that, if they can show "cost-effectiveness," then they are fairly sure of gaining more permanent funding. Their goal is to set up units around the country, and of course to develop their skills as they go.

James Partridge could have written his book and then moved on. Though he wrote that the experience of facial disfigurement never goes away, he could have continued his life as farmer and part-time teacher. In fact, he has drawn on the strength he gained over the years of recovery to aid others in the most massive way, not just in going out and acting as the figurehead and mascot for fund raising, but also in his counseling work, helping many confront their worst times, *his* worst times, again and again, helping many of the 1450 himself, guiding clients through a most painful coming to terms, finding the strength again and again to relive his own experience.

But why Changing Faces, when most of their work is done with people whose faces, for whatever reason, be it burns, cancer, or a congenital problem like cleft lip, cannot be returned to normality by surgery? Changing Faces is about an individual being reconciled to a changed face, being able to develop his or her self-esteem with it and not by ignoring it, for only in this way can such persons step out into the world. Only then can they be aware of others for their own sake, and be seen as an individual, a person, and not as a marker of their own social stigmata or limitations. And the way, possibly the only way, to become reconciled and to rebuild a life is to use not the mirror on the wall but the mirrored perceptions of oneself that others bring.

Merleau-Ponty wrote, "I live in the facial expression of the other, as I feel him living in mine." The whole aim of Changing Faces shows this truth in action. For only by seeking out and meeting people and receiving their reactions to one as a person—not as a facially disfigured being—has the rehabilitation been successful. In fact, as the workshops continue, James has found that many clients have said that a principal reason for coming has been the simple one of learning how to make friends again, to have friends again after their disfigurement.

Changing Faces is really about changing minds. By sending the facially disfigured back into the world, it enriches both their lives and ours: for disfigured people it encourages and enables a fuller life; for the rest of us it gives us all the chance to look below the surface and to concentrate on the person within. For if the facially disfigured are condemned to live in their homes or support groups, we are condemned to lose awareness of the variety of existence. James Partridge wrote, "I have never intentionally used my disfigurement as an excuse . . . I have tried to cultivate the art of wearing my face with pride. Above all my face has opened new doors in my understanding of life and people. I refuse to see it as a handicap."

Fine words. And to meet him is to believe them, and to realize the enormity of his journey for their truth to be earned.

Face Odyssey

12

Maps of Feelings

Go then, friends said, go and talk with the beautiful, using the cover of "researching a book." Seek the famous, known by their faces: royalty, models, TV newscasters, dumb blondes bemoaning their fate to be "just" beautiful. Go look at cosmetic surgery. I could have deplored the need for people to have face-lifts and stave off aging, while defending each person's right to do so, and pointing out how much better such people often feel. I hesitated, not feeling drawn to their experiences. After all, these people have a voice: their stories fill magazines, books, and talk shows the world over; their pictures are everywhere, with little expected beyond their physical perfections.

Instead, I was drawn to those without a voice, to those with something wrong. Those like Mary who had originally blown apart my unthinking conception of the face and personality as one seamless whole. What was it like to live without representation of self externally, and internally, on the face, and not to have the reassurance of others reflecting your worth back to you by their smile? These people seemed to have been forced to an exploration of themselves in a way and to a degree which others had not. I thought once more of Nietzsche writing of illness "halting the unselfconscious flow of life—its ease, its naturalness, its taking everything for granted . . . " In those with facial problems this unselfconscious flow of life had been interrupted, forcing them to consider aspects of the self and of the face not revealed in the glossy magazines.

So I talked with those looking after people with cerebral palsy, who sometimes have no control over their facial and speech muscles. I talked with the doctors and caregivers of those with psychiatric conditions, for there is increasing evidence for disturbances in facial expression and its perception in a wide variety of psychiatric illnesses. Most psychiatric conditions indeed may be seen on the face, but this is not all. Persons with chronic schizophrenia, for instance, may interpret and perceive facial expressions differently—as being more threatening—as well as use facial expressivity and eye contact less.[1] Depressed people may have reduced recognition of affect from faces compared with words.[2] All these altered perceptions of facial expression increase the distance between these people and the rest of us.

I spoke with Alison Muir, a speech therapist, who looked after people, often with no clear diagnosis,[3] who had recently been released from long-term care in large psychiatric hospitals. These persons had limited attention and poor awareness of others, and no social skills, having lived for years in an asocial society. Alison Muir noticed reasonable verbal skills in one man but very poor recognition and use of facial expression. Unable to know what he felt and thought, she began very simply, by sitting with him and showing him facial expressions drawn in cartoon form or in books and magazines. Then with her hands she moved his face to a smile, making him look in a mirror to see a smile, *his* smile, trying to show him for the first time a relation between smiling and happiness. She gave him a set of faces with various expressions, which he called his "maps of feelings." He was by no means unique; Alison saw that most of her clients had impoverished expressions and that they had great difficulty with making appropriate eye contact. She could not know their emotional lives; they had neither the words nor the expressions. One man who had hardly spoken for years reached for his feelings through art, beginning to speak by saying, "Monet's picture is quiet, I feel like the picture."

I went to see a group of deaf people.[4] As they sign they look not at the hands but at the face. Sign language involves an extraordinary fusion of linguistic information from arm movement and facial posturing, as well as the usual affective communication given by facial expression. These nonmanual features help define words and phrases and can give meaning to otherwise ambiguous phrases and sentences. I tried to tease out how deaf people untangled the linguistic use of the face from its emotional use. It proved almost impossible, for though they distinguished the uses effortlessly they found it most difficult to discuss and explain, so deeply was the use of the face in emotional expression buried in them. Despite their loss of sound they took for granted, in a Nietzschean sense, what I was trying to dissect out.

Hearing Emotions, Thinking Emotions

So I went to others who were able to discuss facial matters. In congenitally blind people like Peter White, voice had replaced vision completely in the characterization of others and in their construction of a social world. The face, while allowing some expression, both felt and socially determined, was also important as being where personal attention was focused.[5] Though their world was as richly emotional as ours, there was a suggestion that their range of emotional experience, especially when applied to those they were not intimate with, may be different in subtle ways from our own.

The effortless way in which emotion was revealed to the congenitally blind in voice was exposed by the experience of John Hull. Following his adult onset of blindness, he became engaged in a long struggle to replace his lost visual world of loved ones and colleagues with affective satisfaction and aesthetic pleasure from sound and touch. This journey had revealed much of what the face does for us all. The embedment of face within their minds was evident by the persistent daydreams of faces that both he and Jeremy experienced soon after their blindness. The importance of vision was evident in that their loss of strength after blindness came not when they lost their sight but when they could no longer rely on visual imagery of their friends and family. John described in revelatory detail the passage from a visual engagement with his family and with the world to an auditory and tactile one, something we can scarcely imagine. He felt his very self to be in jeopardy for "to be seen is to exist." Again and again he focused on loss of the revealed person through the face.[6]

If blindness is a world not shared or imagined by sighted people, then autism is an even more private existence, possibly *the* most private existence. Whereas blind people can compare experiences, the idea that autistic persons might communicate or engage and share in social exchange is often out of the question. This makes the preconscious monologues of those exceptionally gifted persons with autism so important. Though the faces of people with autism are hardly remarkable, their use of facial expression and gaze, and their most profound problems with the use of others' faces, brought me directly to the seemingly absolute barrier which they place between themselves and others. The use of the face in those with autism seemed to help toward understanding the condition. And just as faces require free-flowing reciprocities of expression and relatedness—facial conversations—Donna Williams's responses to my questions, by reflection, helped tell how faces define us "typicals," in her terms, "on-line" sentient beings with appropriate "self-other balance."[7]

Autism is a complex developmental neurological problem with few visible external stigmata. In contrast, for people with Möbius syndrome the lack of facial animation is their main and often sole problem and is completely visible, condemning them to be defined by it in the eyes of others. In James and in Clare, though not in all people with Möbius, the absence of expression of emotion through facial movement seemed to have led to an impoverishment of emotions themselves. Mary had not realized her lack of facial expressiveness. Similarly, James was, to a large extent, unaware of the contribution of his facial problem to his feelings of poor self worth. He had been led to a view of his self in which his face played little part, with consequences he was only beginning to explore in his fifties. The facial problem that was so immediate and so obvious to me had been repressed, with his feelings of poor worth being directed to his self, not his face.

A similar story emerged in talking with Clare. She told me that she had never discussed her feelings and experiences with anyone and scarcely explored them herself. She had not the means of making explicit her feelings—no words and no way to feel. She too had not connected her perceptions of low esteem with her face. She too had turned her back on her face years ago, disinvesting in it, living not in her body, not in her face, not in the world, but in her head. A startlingly similar observation was made by Jenny, who had a small facial scar and yet could move her face almost normally. She too was so consumed by her problems that she was hardly aware that they arose from her unusual facial appearance. Others too had made this error. Edward's wife had assumed he was just getting more fixed and grumpy in his old age, not seeing the face for what it was, just for what it expressed. The face seemed invisible, so embedded were her perceptions of it in representing mood, emotion, and self.

Wittgenstein's great book, *Remarks on the Philosophy of Psychology,*[8] was about many matters, but a large part of it was about the relation between what is within us and how it is expressed. For him, as for Peter Hobson, an important part of that was given, instinctive. For Wittgenstein, though not for Hobson so much—the latter's psychoanalytical background led him in a different direction—the face was the interlocutor between the self and the world, and facial action and feeling were intimately linked. Wittgenstein:

"We see emotion."—As opposed to what?—We do not see facial contortions and make the inference that he is feeling joy, grief, boredom. We describe a face immediately as sad, radiant, bored, even when we are unable to give any other description of the features. Grief, one would like to say, is personified in the face. This is essential to what we call "emotion." (p. 570)

The content of an emotion—here one imagines something like a picture. The human face might be called such a picture . . . (p. 148)

A picture, or even moving pictures, however, may be a poor analogy, for the face involves an injunction not only to observe but to immerse oneself in what is expressed. Facial expressions are concerned not only with communication outward but with relatedness and *sharing* of feeling. Hobson:

For a child to perceive a smile as a smile is for the child to be drawn into a quality of relatedness to the smiling person, such that the child is inclined to smile . . . [9]

A smile not associated with positive emotions is not a smile. Wittgenstein:

Would (a) fixed smile really be a smile? And why not?—I might not be able to react as I do to a smile. Maybe it would not make me smile myself. (p. 63)

This immediacy of communication and sharing of emotion from facial expression seem universal, yet they are not something that autistic subjects would recognize, and not part of James's experience. He had related how he *thought* he was in love rather than *felt* it initially, suggesting difficulties in experiencing emotions which may have had their origins in the lack of embodied feeling his Möbius experience imposed.

Once, when talking about these difficulties, James went on to link this with problems in interpreting others.

"I have thought sad . . . I am sad, but do I feel sad as a state of mind and rather than a feeling? I don't think I am very good at reading others' facial movements, so that if someone comes to me sad or happy I don't think I immediately see that person as sad or happy. There is a delay while I work out whether he is coming on happy or sad, at a level of conscious thought."

Contrast this with Hobson who wrote, correctly, that normally

the perception is not a two stage process of which the first stage is the perception of . . . behavioral or bodily form, and the second is an intellectually-based attribution of meaning. Rather the perception is of the meaning itself . . . To perceive a smile is to be inclined to feel certain things.

If imitation allows us to empathize with others, James seems here to be revealing a few of the problems he faced not only in experiencing his own emotions but in sharing them with others.

Controlling Emotions

Parents will have watched their young children having tantrums and rages, especially during the "terrible two's." During this time infants give a full expression to their apparently consuming emotional experience. Slowly, with the months and years, the tantrums subside as the child learns to control expressions of frustration and, one imagines, learns to control the inner feelings themselves. In part this learning is made possible by the effect the child's rages have on others, that is, it has a social dimension. Though studies on children brought up alone are few, they do suggest that these children can move from one emotional state to another quickly and sometimes with little apparent reason.

This evidence suggests a relation between the expression of emotion and learning to control it. This was a recurrent problem for those with Möbius, for Clare and James, as well as the younger Duncan. James was considered very placid and yet this seems a judgment based on his expression, or lack of it, rather than on what he was experiencing. "I have a fear of being out of control with emotions. I would like to be able to cry, but you see I am not really able to."

James talked of no one being available to help until he "dropped the tea tray," that is, broke down, of there being no way of expressing anything before that. Clare found similar problems in expression and control of emotion, but when she couldn't cope she dropped the tray with such power that she was admitted to hospital on several occasions to be restrained.

One might have thought that being bad at expressing emotion might have made one good at controlling it. James controlled so much, and for so long, that in the end the lid came off and he broke down. We seem to need to experience and express strong emotions and to measure the appropriate amount to show and to feel. This learning process may need embodiment of emotional expression in our gestures and facial expression as well as in language, and from studies of feral children and from institutions it also seems to require social regulation from our family and peers.

The other person afraid of losing emotional control was Donna Williams, who defined her autism as being, at its core, an emotional disorder. It is scarcely possible to analyze the interactions between the inability to process information into meaning and the emotional and ontological problems associated with autism. But what does seem possible is that in some autistic people the lack of coherent emotional expression and selfhood, coupled with their asocial existence, leaves them at risk of emotional lack of control which may be made apparent by severe behavioral outbursts.

Measuring Skulls

The more I delved into research on the subject the more there seemed to be an implicit relationship between the development of the face and of the mind, both in evolutionary terms and in human development. In parallel with this, from the narratives of those with facial dysfunction it was apparent that they shared particular problems in emotional experience and in their social existence. These questions—of mind, of emotion, of sociability, and of embodiment—seem to coalesce at the face.

In 1971 the psychologist Nick Humphrey found himself, as a student of Dian Fossey, measuring skulls of gorillas killed by poachers in Rwanda. He would go out to watch groups of gorillas in the jungle, and began to wonder why their skulls and brains were so large when all they did was wander around eating, sleeping and playing.

I had come to Africa not primarily for scientific reasons, but to escape from an impossible human situation at home . . . My head (when I was not thinking about gorillas) was full of unresolved problems concerning my social relationships. Suddenly I saw the animals with new eyes. I realized that, for them too, their problems were probably primarily social ones . . .

. . . Life in the forest seems to pose so few problems for these apes precisely because the gorilla family, as a social unit, is so well adapted to it . . . A gorilla infant does not have to discover what is good or bad to eat; his mother teaches him.

The problems of creating and maintaining such a stable group are quite another matter. They know each other intimately, they know their place. Nonetheless there are endless small disputes about social dominance. . . .

The intelligence required to survive socially is something of a quite different order to that needed to cope with the material world. Social intelligence is clearly the key to the great ape's biological success.[10] (pp. 18–19)

The evolution of the primates is a complex and multifaceted story, with climatic and dietary changes and many other factors playing their parts. But one reason for primates' successful development may have been because their social groupings became dependent on interpersonal relationships in a way completely different from the huge impersonal yet exquisitely structured colonies of ants or bees. This might have required not just simple predictions about behavior, but insight into another's feelings. The cognitive skill needed for servicing such groups is considerable, for as group size increases, apes must understand and remember a large number of relationships. This is particularly true for groups with leisure time to interact, for example, chimpanzees. Large groups are unstable unless the individual relationships within the groups are serviced regularly and large complex groups need large complex brains.

One index of social intelligence in primates might be the average size of the elementary social group of a species. Dunbar has provided evidence that relative brain size in primates increases with the size of the social groups they form.[11] Complexity of behavior means a movement away from simple stimulus-reward reflexes, to a weighing up of options both in relation to the external situation and in relation to memory of the past and to the internal mental state of the individual. More complex and subtle behavior appears to involve unpredictability of mood and needs the recognition of various internal states in another.[12] How are relationships between animals to be maintained? How are the ties of dominance and submission and of kinship to be recognized?

Language probably evolved too late to influence this development of social intelligence. As our early social groupings became more subtle and complexities of social display increased, expression of inner states depended on early vocalization and on body language. In primates this gestural language moved from being a whole body thing to being expressed and elaborated on the face. Facial, as opposed to postural, emotional expression becomes more important in the most highly evolved primates. Monkeys usually combine a facial expression with a postural signal. In anthropoid apes facial expression is more independent of posture. Finally, in humans, facial expression emerges as a modality on its own.

The development of a more complex social structure may have required the development of "mind" to serve it. And this "mind," or intelligence, did not develop initially as a memory bank, or cognitive intelligence, to locate food or water, but as a social intelligence, which enabled the relationships between individuals upon which our ancestors' evolutionary success depended. Individuality in this sense may have been a new evolutionary concept. With this came more highly evolved faces which provided both the unique identifier of each animal, and the way in which each individual's mind state could be determined and communicated. As the face became more mobile and articulate, the emotional language itself may have been refined too.[13]

Once our ancestors developed language, previously unimaginable levels of abstract thought and cognitive intelligence emerged. But before this, the evolution of the social groupings upon which our success depended, and our development of social intelligence and emotional expression, are difficult to conceive of without the parallel evolution of face.[14]

No Different Today

The evolution of the face, of complex groups, and of social intelligence itself might therefore be linked. But surely with the development of language and our huge increase in brain size and power there has been a downgrading in the importance of the affective mind. Today are we not driven less by desire and emotion and more by rational thought and cognitive deduction?

Recently, Antonio Damasio has shown how important emotion is to our functioning in all aspects of everyday life.[15] Drawing on patients with brain damage in the frontal lobes, in whom affective feelings have been reduced or abolished, he has shown that such individuals may have normal intelligence and memory, even normal powers of rational problem solving, but are unable to exist normally in the world. They cannot make decisions about even some everyday matters, since decisions require both information and an emotional feeling toward something to come down on one side or another.[16] Such patients also lose perception of others so that they have little interpersonal relatedness, a loss of theory of mind unrelated to autism.

Those areas of the brain Damasio suggested were necessary for the processing of emotion and its input to decision making include the amygdala and inferofrontal cortex, areas similar to those suggested by Simon Baron-Cohen to be associated with eye-direction detection and the theory-of-mind mechanism, and by others to be involved in face processing as a whole. These areas of the brain are large enough to have several functions, but the overlapping anatomy is striking.

Damasio distinguished between emotions—internal mind states and feelings—and their expression in the body, and suggested varieties of feelings. The first followed emotions and were the sort that Paul Ekman suggested are "basic" because they are shown unambiguously and universally on the face—happiness, anger, disgust, fear. When the body, including the face, moves in a way that conforms to these profiles, we feel the emotion. More subtle emotions are variations on the themes of basic emotions: euphoria, ecstasy, and wistfulness, for example, and are tuned by experience, "when subtler shades of cognitive state are connected to subtler variations of emotional body state." Lastly, background feelings correspond to the states existing most of the time between emotions—"the body landscape when not shaken by emotion."

Being aware of one's emotional state, Damasio suggests, allows flexibility of response based on a personal history of interactions with the environment. Feelings are felt via the brain and through feedback from the body, not just the face. Feedback from the body means feelings secondary to changes in blood flow and patterns of activation of skin, gut and muscle, which we learn to associate with certain emotions.[17] He paints a picture of the importance of internal feedback for our comparing emotions in differing situations.

Feelings are sensors for the match or lack thereof between nature and circumstance. Feelings, along with the emotions they come from, are not a luxury. They are the result of a most curious physiological arrangement that has turned the brain into the body's captive audience. (p. xv)

Damasio reaffirms the deep and essential embodiment that our emotional lives depend on, so questioning Descartes' separation of mind and body.

William James and James

Damasio's thesis echoes and extends that of William James—that an emotion depends on and *is* its bodily expression.[18] What Damasio does not discuss in such detail is the need to communicate feelings to others. While language may do this, it is not good at the expression of emotion and feelings. Autonomic expressions of emotion, the racing heart or clammy hands of extreme fear, do not communicate either. Emotions are revealed and experienced through the body and especially in humans, the face. Even Damasio's "background feelings" may be expressed on our faces. How often are we greeted by someone who, on seeing our countenance, asks if we feel a certain mood, which we do, even though we had hardly been aware of it?

Such feedback, of course, is not limited to our own feelings from our body. More important for our social existence and self-esteem perhaps is the feedback from others. Aspects of our very being may be defined by others. As Merleau-Ponty wrote, "I live in the facial expression of the other, as I feel him living in mine."

This truth was shown again and again in those with facial problems. Their unusual faces prevented any reflection, in the facial expression of others, which did not reinforce their separateness and alienation. For example, Changing Faces seeks to give people with facial problems other avenues of expression and to give them the means to manage social interactions independently of their faces, as individuals with personal gifts to offer, not as people defined by their stigma.

We may now see how the various and apparently haphazard collection of case histories and narratives in this book are related. The different categories of problems, sensory as in blindness, physical as in facial disfigurement and Möbius, neurological as in Bell's palsy, and developmental as in autism—some congenital, some experienced later in life—collapse, blur, and overlap at the face. For all these case histories tell of the disconnection between mind and body in a very specific way, between that part of mind concerned with emotion and its elaboration in the face.

They tell of difficulties in the calibration and experience of emotion and in the essential deeply embedded role of the face in our perception of self and of soul. Their profound difficulties in a social existence keep returning us to the crucial part that existence plays in our well being. All tell of the essential role of the face in the expression and experience of feeling itself. Those who were hardly aware of the facial origin of their problems show how deep within us are these matters that they are only brought to light by a shattering disconnection between personality and the face; this was what Mary's case revealed instantly to me.

Autism, of course, is not a facial problem in the way Möbius syndrome is. Despite these differences, those with Möbius have, at times, been labeled autistic because their facial immobility has prevented normal social interaction and emotional expression. Those in long-term psychiatric care show similar autistic features.[19] In the workshops at Changing Faces one of the most difficult things is to get people with facial disfigurement to look other people in the face. Their facial problems have led to an almost autistic withdrawal from others. There is even beginning to be evidence for delay in the development of symbolic play, sharing behavior, and the use of first-person pronouns like "I" and "me" in congenitally blind children, who lack the ability to see the relatedness of another and so cannot calibrate their feelings from other's faces.[20]

If emotions need expression through feelings in the body, it follows that a lack of experience of feeling from the face may lead to a reduced ability for emotional experience itself. Oliver, with the Bell's palsy, described being in an emotional limbo, not knowing what he felt, and resorted to a diary to write down and try to reach his emotions.

It becomes clear from those who have lost facial animation how crucial facial embodiment is for our emotional existence. One could even legitimately ask, Why, when we talk of "embodiment," is there no term for this crucial facial embodiment? Is it because, as for Mary and for James, it is so obvious we cannot see it? James, "the spectator," who has never known such embodiment, described a curious detachment, *thinking* he was happy rather than feeling it. Without feelings from the face emotions may be less clearly defined and so less fully experienced, and James was less able to enter the full presence of others. I once said to him that seeing others and seeing how they felt was the beginning of relating to them. He replied, "I have not tried to think about how they feel. I have not done this by looking. Communication for me began with the words. It was language and by thought that my relationship was formed."

In the beginning was the Word, for James as for Saint John, and for Freud in psychoanalysis. Yet for most of us the word, the theory, the intellect, is not the beginning. We engage and gain experience in an emotional domain dependent on the face and feelings.

Oliver mentioned that he could not lie on the phone. Sometimes we all use words to conceal while knowing our faces are telling another story. When these counterpoints and harmonies between different channels and levels of communication were no longer possible, clarity of expression seemed more important for him. We should not, perhaps, think of the different channels for expression (facial, vocal, and body language) as being separate; they seem to require and depend on one another. For instance, those with Parkinson's found that when their faces were more animated, their voices became so too, over the phone and in everyday living. Edward's wife described how he came alive again in many ways once he found a way to improve facial animation.

Phantom Emotions

Donna Williams told me that as a child she had emotions but no feelings. Many of her bizarre movements and actions, even, say, tapping a finger, were attempts to express emotion, but could not be seen as such by others. Much of what Donna seems to be exploring in her writing is the way in which she grew up with emotions but with no ability to map them onto experience, or onto feelings, either in herself or in others. She describes this lack of embodiment:

I still do not feel right with the idea that I am my body, I have had the experience of this but it is not consistent. Mostly I think I exist in my sub-conscious or pre-conscious mind . . . [21]

Children with congenitally absent arms and legs may still experience phantom limb sensations. Within the brain, innately, there appear to be areas concerned with limb perception, even though they never join onto the sensory experiences coming from the arm or leg and so never become embodied. In autism there may be areas of "phantom emotion" which may be similarly innate, yet disconnected with, and uncalibrated by, experiences and feelings from self and from others. In Möbius, though such phantom emotions have not been described, it seems that full emotional lives may be hampered by a lack of embodied feeling and reflected feeling. Mapping facial expressions and feelings in the appropriate social situation onto inner and innate emotions may be one of the many complex tasks children do in their early years.

This leads to the question as to why congenitally blind people learn so well to compensate for their lack of shared facial expressiveness whereas some of those with Möbius do not (recall that most persons with Möbius do well socially and are happy with their situation). It may be, in part, that the blind do express emotion facially (though they use their faces less, socially), and experience their own facial animation in the appropriate situations in a way that people with Möbius cannot. Possibly the blind enter a culture that is aware of them and that can cope with the additional needs of blind children.

But a different explanation presents itself from the experience of Jenny, whose facial scar she felt was unsightly but whose facial expressiveness was normal, and from many others with facial disfigurements. There may be such a stigma attached to having an unusual face that social interaction and emotional engagement are not initiated by others. An individual may be surrounded by others and yet be alone. That is why I wondered earlier what sort of life people with Möbius would have enjoyed in a community of the blind, and that is why the work of James Partridge and those at Changing Faces is so important. Whichever explanation is correct, social skills and facial games can be taught, and such people helped.

Face Value

Gender, age, mood, character, health, tiredness, attractiveness—so much is taken in from a glance at someone else's face. Yet usually in our social relations we do not look at people but exchange glances or share a mutual gaze. And in so doing we experience another in a more extensive and intimate way than does a chimpanzee viewing a fellow chimpanzee. We see and feel emotion, we see and relate to another individual. The more we look into another mind, the more that involves engagement between individuals. Caroline Garland had said that, as a psychoanalyst, she was trying the whole time to think of what sort of a person she was for the other person, trying the whole time to see herself from another's viewpoint.

When we look into another's eyes the experience of the other is more than a series of thoughts, intents, desires, or concealments. These may be present but, more than these, we expose our emotions to the world too. Some of these aspects have been considered by the French philosopher Emmanuel Levinas.[22] For Levinas the uniqueness of the face is that it always remains the face of another, and so cannot be assimilated fully into oneself. I always see a face as foreign, and this foreign-ness means that it cannot be fully comprehended or encompassed. If the face—meaning another's face—remains foreign, then it becomes evident that it is beyond my full grasp or control. The expression of the other, in terms of speech as well as facial movement, does two things: it gives a message I can comprehend, but it also signifies something beyond the comprehension—in terms of being able to be explained. Much of art is attempting to understand and communicate this, as, in another context, is psychoanalysis.

For Levinas it follows that there is something in the human face-to-face relationship that I, as subjective ego, cannot control, and insofar as it disrupts my control, my ego, it puts me into question or jeopardy. The "putting into question" that facial relationships involve was seen in the Changing Faces workshops and in the stories of those with Möbius. But it has never been expressed better than by those with autism. Donna Williams wrote in response to my suggestion of seeing her paintings,

I have no idea what you could take from my art. I have a momentary panic that you even consider the concept of taking from me (for it IS me externalised in color and form on paper). Yet this shouldn't surprise me—it was that same sense of others' taking from experiencing my expression that kept my expression hidden and un-shared for so many years—just not quite grasped like right now. Anyway, logically, I have considered that you can't ACTUALLY take anything away because the pictures will stay here.

If face-to-face relationships involve feelings toward and between people, any external face, another's face, puts a demand on me. It asks me to recognize another, for what I cannot fully assimilate I must respect, and for Levinas this recognition summons me to a form of moral responsibility, in the face of the other, which cannot be brought under the control of my reason and therefore cannot be explained. This moral or ethical responsibility can be viewed in terms of the need for a response, for the face of the other requires me to respond and enter into a relationship, but a relationship I cannot fully control, that neither of us can fully control. It involves a risk so evident for many of those with facial problems that they avoid it.

Theory of Mind?

My personal feeling—my internal, scarcely conscious, emotional intuition—was that a subjective exploration of facial problems was required, as well as an objective account of various aspects of face. This I hope I have achieved to a small degree, though it has not always been easy to enter, or share, or at least seek to understand, different worlds. I have felt at times like a psychiatrist who takes on board his patients' problems, since any attempt to understand seems to include entering into the experience of others. In doing this I was concerned about any reluctance on the part of the subjects themselves. On the whole the reverse was the case. People, once they were satisfied as to my probity and sympathetic approach, were pleased that someone was prepared to listen and understand after all these years. The exception was Donna Williams, for whom any attempt by another to understand her autistic world threatened her fragile monotrack sense of self.

So why do I comply with these questions without want or like—merely because it did not occur to me to do something else at the time (for which I generally need cues and at the moment your letter was the only thing cueing me). Do I resent you for this? I've become complacent because it is such a way of life. Part of me has a spark of resentment for it. I kept having the sentence-thought "naughty person" (it is an echoed phrase) when I looked at your pages after a break. If that's an indication, it probably means that some part of me considers your thirst for information to be selfish. Yet, logically, I've learned that non-autistic people generally can't imagine CAN-based action in the absence of like or want [i.e., cannot imagine action without emotion] so in that sense you aren't responsible/culpable for your actions.

When I saw Donna I tried to explain that what "typicals" do is want to imagine other minds, enter other minds, understand other minds. My interest was therefore typical of, and almost defined "typicals."

Her commentary on David's testament showed her to be able to understand the functioning of another autistic person. She might therefore have had some "theory of mind" for another autistic subject. In fact, she seemed to need a theory for what most of us do intuitively. Through her books and then our correspondence I had gained some little understanding of her and Paul's world, but she little of ours, and she was not able to extend her creative act to interpreting beyond David's world. In this the gap between autism and typicals was revealed, for without a sufficiently secure sense of self none of us can imagine others and absorb their experience into our own. That, rather than the world of the blind, is truly an existence without "face."

When she read this section Donna marked it with a tick. "Yes, 'Face' in the real sense of identity or mind." This made me think of what she had written previously in answering my questions:

Where did I reside, if not in my body? My body was often experienced as external and other . . . Sometimes my brain handled everything until my mind was redundant . . . Sometimes, I had emotions without mind. Sometimes, I had pure logic (mind) without emotion.

Yes, the extinguishing of self merely because of the experience of others saddens me too.

Being mono [the experience of being able to keep hold of one system or thing at once] makes it hard to hold simultaneous sense of self (internal feedback and reflection) and other (externally generated information requiring processing).

Seeing Consciousness

"The extinguishing of self merely because of the experiencing of others." Buried in this was the implication that the awareness of self was related to something given by others.

Premack and Woodruff defined theory of mind as imputing mental states to oneself and to others, inferring knowledge, belief, doubt, pretending, and so forth. It was a "theory" because these states could not be known directly. Baron-Cohen, in his elegant exposition of the theory, focused on the importance of the eyes for mind reading, mentioning eye movement detection, shared attention, pupil size, and eyelid position. The face holds a central place in his theories, but mainly, it seems, as a carrier for the eyes.

For Andrew Meltzoff the face is seen more as a whole, so that it is through active facial movement that learning about others and self may be possible. For Peter Hobson, too, one has the impression of the face as a gestalt. What comes first for him is not a cognitive theory construction, but rather an enveloping innate desire for interpersonal relatedness. The first internal states are not intellectual but those that have to do with feelings seen in the actions of others, and in their faces: "Children's understanding of unobservable mental states is not so mysterious once one sees that they begin by understanding mental states that are observable."

These differing theories are not, of course, mutually exclusive. Meltzoff's focus is upon very early development, in the first few hours and days and months of life. At that time innate facial imitation may have the crucial role. Hobson, in looking at interpersonal relatedness, seems to be considering early infancy. His work may point toward a possible way in which later cognitive strategies for interpersonal skill and social manipulation emerge. Later in development, such theories of mind may be more important and this research has proved very useful in looking at development.

The *Oxford English Dictionary* gives its first illustrative citation of "being conscious" as, "knowing something with others, knowing in oneself" (1601). In discussing theory of mind and interpersonal relationships we have been skirting carefully round questions about consciousness. For if consciousness does depend on awareness of others, and perhaps of our own feelings, then it is difficult to imagine its development without the evolution of the face, for often when we see someone thinking or feeling we have the impression of seeing consciousness.

The intimacy between the face, emotion and consciousness was discussed by Merleau-Ponty in *Phenomenology and the Sciences of Man.*[23] "What is it to be moved, what is the meaning of emotion? Can one conceive of a consciousness which is incapable of emotion?" Further on he suggests that "The relation of language to thought is [here] comparable to that of the body to consciousness." I would suggest that the word "face" replace "body" in this sentence, as did the great Scottish physiologist Charles Bell: ". . . the thought is to the word as the feeling is to the face."[24] Here consciousness is thought to arise from—and be embedded in—the body. More than that, it is thought to exist—and possibly originate—in an emotional domain. This may have begun in mammals and primates by attention to, and awareness of, internal states of autonomic arousal, like flight and fright, which Damasio discusses, but it was successfully elaborated to higher levels of emotional refinement and awareness in parallel with the evolution of the face. In this it may have been driven by internal factors of expression and experience, but also by a social dimension. Merleau-Ponty went on to stress that "the intellectual elaboration of our experience of the world is constantly supported by the affective elaboration of our inter-human relations."

Go back to the work on primates; the elaboration of more refined faces proceeded with more complex social groups and, possibly, to the beginnings of awareness itself. Recall the most intelligent monkeys, the bonobos; recall their mobile faces and acceptance of prolonged mutual gaze.

If indeed it is difficult to imagine consciousness without the face and facial animation, that is not to say that the face reveals inner mind states simply or uniformly. Each person has a different countenance and facial habits, and the way in which each of us interprets these may differ too. Merleau-Ponty: "I seize the other's psyche only indirectly . . . mediated by its body appearances. I cannot know what you are thinking, but I can guess at it from your facial expression." These guesses depend on knowing the person you are engaged with and the context. But note the element of guessing. If through faces we interpret others, then these interpretations are not precise. Rather they inhabit a world of the preconscious, which we are aware of and act on, but find difficult to describe.

Each of us may take something slightly different from a person—frequently people disagree about what a person is "like" even when they have seen him or her at the same time—because these interpretations depend on imagination which in turn is related to the experience of a person and each person's creativity.

Looking into others' minds—feeling toward others—is not a precise science but requires imagination and creativity. It is perhaps the most creative thing we do each day, as we seek to match faces with characters and personal experiences. That was what Jeremy, the recently blind man, was trying to do when giving new acquaintances the faces of old friends in his imagination. Perhaps the very origins of our creativity lie in our compulsive desire to look into the faces of others.[25]

The Divine Fantasy

Our facial movements include those both ancient and modern. Some are common to other primates, like an enjoyment smile. Some, like the Elvis snarl, are unique to our species. Some may have evolved in a fairly simple way from protective reflexes, while others have been adopted more recently to express emotion and feeling, social purpose, and inner states. Though we and the other primates evolved from a common ancestor millions of years ago, we can recognize some similarity in facial display between ourselves and chimpanzees and gorillas, and not only in facial display but in their relation to behavior and even mood.

Part six-million-year-old display rule predictor, part emotion readout, part cultural, part innate, part conscious, part not, the face is, in Duchenne's words, a "divine fantasy" and we will remain fascinated and enraptured by its movements as long as we remain interested in one another as individuals. In Mao's China personal mirrors were banned for being bourgeois.[26]

Liggett wrote:

Maybe the time is not too far distant when the equations linking face and character will be written with certainty. We must await the development of an entirely new technology of facial description and analysis which matches in power and precision the science of personality. Then we shall be able to pronounce with certainty on the relationship of face and character."[27]

May those days be far away, for face and facial expression define our uniqueness and individuality and act to conceal as well as to reveal. We would be exposed and threatened if the intimacy we allow a few were to be available to all. The face fascinates in part by its mystery and by our creative acts at interpretation.

So, in the end, the face is involved in theory of mind and the development of social intelligence as a precursor to higher cognitive function, and even perhaps to consciousness. But before our intellectual and cognitive selves develop, we begin our lives with innate needs for emotional relatedness without which other development is slowed. In connection with this we spend our early days and years, in part, elaborating use of the face. John Hull describes his daughter groping toward an understanding of this relatedness and its dependence on the face. His diary entry of 21 March 1986 reads:

Yesterday morning I was kneeling on the floor helping Lizzie [aged four] get dressed. When she had finished I stood her up and said,

"Now! Let's have a look at you."

I held her face lightly between my hands, and gave her a big smile.

"Daddy, how can you smile between you and me when I smile and when you smile because you are blind?" I laughed.

"What do you mean, darling. How can I what? With great hesitation she said,

"How can you smile—no—how can I smile between you and me—no—between you and me a smile, when you're blind?"

"You mean, how do I know when to smile at you?"

"Yes."

"It's true, darling, that blind people often don't know when to smile. But today I knew you were smiling, darling, because you were standing there, and I was smiling at you, and I thought you were probably smiling at me. Were you?"

Happily she replied,

"Yes!"

Note that she talked of *a* smile, *a single* smile going between them, a union through feeling through the face to love.

Our intelligence, compared even with that of other primates, may be immense. Our problem solving abilities, powers of abstract thought, our awareness and consciousness are all of apparently different orders of magnitude from those of other animals. We, as a species, have been characterized in the past by our cognitive abilities, by our refined consciousness, by language, by our use of tools, even by our self-destructiveness. Yet we are also unique in that most simple of behaviors, by our compulsion to look each other in the face. In this is revealed our innate desire to enter into other minds, and our intense social being, which may have allowed our evolutionary leap from other primates. Our species may almost be defined by our inquisitiveness about others' lives and minds and thoughts.

With these, perhaps coming before them, may have been a feeling toward others and the entering into relationships. For it is difficult to imagine mind and consciousness without feelings, and feelings without the social and personal communication and definition which the face provides.

This book, then, finally, is about the looking into others and the feeling for—and understanding of—those around us that the face allows, enables, and even requires. I have in turn sought to understand those who, for whatever reason, have learned to exist "without face," for in their narratives, I believe, lies a mirror allowing us all to learn more about face.

"Tell," Mary tapped out on her typewriter, "Tell, please."

I have tried.

Notes

Chapter 1

1. A friend said that it had always amazed him that the mad or sad *looked* mad or sad, and it is amazing. Just a glance at a depressed person, for instance, reveals how they are.

2. Kurt Goldstein, *The Organism,* New York: Zone Books, 1995.

3. The face obviously cannot be taken in isolation from other communication channels like the voice and the body (see below), but while language and gesture have been the object of many excellent studies, some of these aspects of the face have not been considered in detail. See David MacNeill, *Hand and Mind.* Chicago: Chicago University Press, 1992, and Steven Pinker, *The Language Instinct.* New York: William Morrow, 1994; London: Penguin Press, 1994.

4. One case similar to Mary's has been described, though there must be more. This patient had much more sudden loss of facial movement and swallowing which was traced to strokes on both sides of the brain. See M. W. L. Chee, C. B. Tan, and H. T. L. Tjia, "Persistent mutism and dysphagia of acute onset due to bilateral internal capsule infarction," *Annals of the Academy of Medicine* 19 (1990): 393–395.

Chapter 2

1. It is not true, of course, to say that blind people do not receive feedback of what their face is doing. They still have the internal feedback of movement and touch of the face. Blind children soon learn the effect their expression has on others and learn to respond accordingly. Where this does not happen is in feral children (children apparently living their early years without the company of other humans, the so-called wolf children), and there are few data on their refinement of facial expression.

2. Peter White spoke truer than he may have known. There is beginning to be a large literature on the way in which brain function may alter after injury, repudiating earlier work suggesting that no change occurred in brains after injury. Those with congenital blindness seem to have brains given over more to hearing and touch, while congenitally deaf people have areas of the brain normally involved in the analysis of some aspects of hearing altered to be responsive to visual and tactile information. Such plastic changes in the brain seem larger if damage to normal function occurs early in life. In those in whom brain injury occurs as adults, the extent of functional recovery, and hence of presumed plastic change, may be less and may depend on the motivational state of the individual. Two recent source papers on plasticity and much else are V. S. Ramachandran, "Behavioural and magnetoencephalographic correlates of plasticity in the adult human brain," *Proceedings of the National Academy of Sciences of the United States of America* 90 (1993): 10413–10420; and V. S. Ramachandran, "Phantom limbs, neglect syndromes, repressed memories and Freudian psychology, *International Review of Neurobiology* 37 (1994): 291–333.

3. The nineteenth-century anatomist, surgeon, and physiologist; see later chapters.

4. Milan Kundera, *Immortality*. New York: Grove Weidenfeld, 1991.

5. An individual's blindness is imposed on an organism which has evolved over many generations with vision. Whether or not the idea of the face would be important if equally intelligent but blind organisms had evolved is another matter. In subsequent chapters I discuss mammalian evolution of the face. These arguments apply to terrestrial mammals. The large aquatic mammals may have developed in a different way.

6. See K. R. Scherer, and H. G. Walbott, "Evidence for universality and cultural variation of differential emotion response patterning," *Journal of Personal and Social Psychology* 66 (1994): 310–328 [with addendum in volume 67, 55]; and V. C. Tartter, and D. Braun, "Hearing smiles and frowns in normal and whisper speech," *Journal of the Acoustical Society of America* 168 (1994): 320–324. I am very grateful to an anonymous MIT reader for bringing these two works to my attention.

Chapter 3

1. John Hull, *Touching the Rock: An Experience of Blindness*. New York: Random House, 1992. This book has been translated into a number of languages.

2. It is not completely clear here if Hull is considering his relationship with his own face and self or those of others. For to some extent my own face, as seen by me and usually mirror-reversed, may have a more elusive and complex image to me than that of other people. When I think of myself I think of what I have done, or am about to do, and my personal "face-self" hardly appears. When I think of others, however, faces are very important. Nor can I be sure that the face I see as myself, with its mirror reversal and self-regarding look, is similar to the image that our friends and loved ones have. It is very difficult to know, even with photography

and, more recently, video. (I am very grateful to Shaun Gallagher for the development and discussion of some of these ideas.)

3. Here Hull is describing the lack of commensurality between perception of a face seen and touched. There does not appear to be any equivalence between the two, perhaps not surprising since we rarely seek to learn faces through touching others.' Rather we know others' faces from sight. Our own we see from photography and so forth and by feeling it internally—these two do not always appear commensurate.

4. Or of other blind people. Both Peter White and David Blunkett did not find, as congenitally blind people, that their worlds were devoid of anything or intellectually clearer than that of their sighted colleagues.

Chapter 4

1. In evolutionary terms human evolution split from that of the other existing primates over four million years ago. There are obvious limitations in thinking that the nonhuman primates reveal what we were like at some earlier and ill defined time.

2. Abnormalities of fusion lead to cleft lip and palate.

3. W. K. Gregory, and G. Lightoller, quoted in J. A. R. A. M. Van Hooff, "The facial displays of catarrhine monkeys and apes." In *Primate Ethology*, edited by D. Morris. London: Weidenfeld & Nicholson, 1967.

4. In 1772 Johann Caspar Lavater published *Essays on Physiognomy, Physiognomical Fragments of the Promotion of the Knowledge and Love of Mankind*. This massive work on judging interior reality by external appearance had soon gone to sixteen German, fifteen French, two American, and twenty English versions. The book mixes ideas about facial expression, with which we might agree, with "facts" about form that we could not, for example, "a flat somewhat sinking forehead denotes an unpolished person confined within a small circle of domestic economy." The neck was considered to give evidence of sincerity; the nose and cheeks, morality.

5. One man asked a surgeon to reduce what he thought were large jaw and forehead bones, since they gave people an impression of an aggressive and unpleasant face, at odds with his true personality. His life was altered after realignment of his facial bones made him appear less aggressive. He found, for instance, that people were friendlier and kinder to him and that all aspects of social interaction were easier. His surgeon called this the "Minotaur syndrome." See P. G. Morselli, "The Minotaur syndrome: Plastic surgery of the facial skeleton," *Aesthetic Plastic Surgery* 17 (1993): 99–102.

6. Duchenne thought that some expressions depended on the action of single muscles, though usually more than one muscle is involved in a given expression. Ekman and Friesen describe one such facial action unit, action unit 17, as going from the lower lip to far down the chin. It acts to pull up the skin of the chin and pull the down lower lip, and may wrinkle the chin boss or depress under the lower lip to produce a glum mouth, or to protrude the lower lip, depending on its strength of

activation and the activation of other action units at the time. See P. Ekman, and W. V. Friesen, "Measuring facial movement," *Environmental Psychology and Nonverbal Behaviour* 1 (1976): 56–75. A recent review by Ekman of his work may be found in P. Ekman, Facial expression of emotion: An old controversy and new findings. In *Processing the Facial Image,* edited by V. Bruce et al. 63–69. Oxford: Clarendon Press, 1992.

7 . Though some recovery of muscle function commonly occurs after damage to other nerves, this recovery rarely leads to obvious synkinesis. It is not clear if this is because facial nerve innervation is so much more obvious than that of other muscles (for it is displayed on the face), or because facial nerve innervation is more exquisitely selective in the muscles individual nerve fibers go to.

8. Ekman has suggested that the outside of the orbital muscle cannot be contracted voluntarily into a smile.

9. See G. B. Duchenne, *The Mechanism of Human Facial Expression or an Electro-Physiological Analysis of the Expression of the Emotions,* translated by A. Cuthbertson. 1862. Reprint New York: Cambridge University Press, 1990.

10. S. Arroyo et al., "Mirth, laughter and gelastic seizures," *Brain* 116 (1993): 757–780.

11. One study found ninety percent recognition of photos of classmates (from 90 to 900 in number) between three months and thirty-five years later. See H. P. Bahrick, O. O. Bahrick, and R. P. Wittlinger, "Fifty years of memory for names and faces: a cross sectional approach," *Journal of Experimental Psychology: General* 104 (1975): 54–75. Recognition of faces increases steadily in children with age. Interestingly, there is a small fall-off with adolescence as, perhaps, attention is turned inward more.

12. Oliver Sacks, *The Man Who Mistook His Wife for a Hat.* New York: Summit, 1985.

13. J. Sergent, and J.-L. Signoret, "Functional and anatomical decomposition of face processing: Evidence from prosopagnosia and PET study of normal subjects." *Philosophical Transactions of the Royal Society of London. Series B: Biological Sciences* 335 (1992): 55–62. Good reviews are to be found in V. Bruce et al., eds., *Processing the Facial Image,* Oxford: Clarendon Press, 1992. This is a collection of papers from the Royal Society meeting at which Sergent and Signoret first presented their paper. More recent papers include, A. W. Young et al., "Face processing impairments after amygdalotomy," *Brain* 118 (1995): 15–24; and J. J. Evans et al., "Progressive prosopagnosia associated with selective right temporal lobe atrophy, *Brain* 118 (1995): 1–13.

14. D. H. Jacobs et al., "Emotional facial imagery, perception and expression in Parkinson's disease," *Neurology* 45 (1995): 1695–1702.

15. It is coming to be recognized that a crucial aspect of face processing is recognition of the direction of gaze of the face observed. This has important implications for social interaction, for one needs to know if the person is looking at you.

Chapter 5

1. Quoted in J. A. Russell, "Is there universal recognition of emotion from facial expression? A review of cross-cultural studies," *Psychological Bulletin* 115 (1994): 102–141.

2. Charles Bell, *Essays on the Anatomy and Physiology of Expression,* 2nd rev. ed., London: John Murray, 1824. Sir Charles Bell was a great early nineteenth-century Scottish anatomist, physiologist, surgeon, and artist. A similar differentiation between emotion and feeling has been proposed by Antonio Damasio in his book *Descartes' Error;* see chapter 11.

3. G. B. Duchenne, *The Mechanism of Human Facial Expression of an Electro-Physiological Analysis of the Expression of the Emotions,* translated by A. Cuthbertson, 1982. Reprint New York: Cambridge University Press, 1990. Guillaume Benjamin Amand Duchenne was a nineteenth-century French physician and neurologist. His most famous description was of the eponymous muscular dystrophy derived from his name. Duchenne also realized how the expression of the entire face could be changed by movement of only one or a few muscles. This led him to suggest that we normally view the face as a gestalt, with a change in a small part of it altering our perception of the whole, something more widely accepted now. He saw that even at repose or between movements there was activity in the muscles that is only lost, "with life itself."

4. Charles Darwin, *The Expression of the Emotions in Man and Animals.* Chicago: University of Chicago Press, 1965. In his book he acknowledges a Mr. Dyson Lace, who made valuable observations several hundred miles in the interior of Queensland. The Reverend Stack observed Maoris in New Zealand and Raja Brooke, the Dyaks of Borneo. The list goes on, with receipt of observations on Chinese immigrants in Malaysia, on the Chinese in China, on Indians from a Mr. Irskin—who had great difficulty owing to the "natives' habitual concealment of emotion from Europeans"—and a Mrs. Barber, who observed the Kafers and Fingoes of Africa.

5. William Montgomery, "Charles Darwin's thought on expressive mechanisms in evolution." In *The Development of Expressive Behavior,* edited by Gail Zivin, 27–50. New York: Academic Press, 1985.

6. In trying to learn why Darwin made such an uncharacteristic suggestion I first asked Richard Dawkins. He referred me to Helena Cronin at the London School of Economics, who in turn passed me on to Paul Ekman, who suggested I read Montgomery. I think Darwin underestimated cultural effects on preadaptation (Dawkins's memes). If he had stressed our social existence more, the evolution of such elaborate facial expressions would not have surprised him. Just how altered behavior might enter the genome remains unclear, though one possible explanation is the Baldwin effect (J. M. Baldwin, "A new factor in evolution," *American Naturalist* 30 (1896): 441–451, 536–553). Baldwin suggested that through learning and shared culture any new and advantageous behavior will soon become available to many. Those who can learn it easily will then be favored by natural selection. Perhaps those babies who learned to smile early were cared for better, and thus were more

likely to survive. Perhaps those adults with genes facilitating smiling and the reception of smiles were selected for in parallel.

7. Paul Ekman has written much on this topic. Two useful texts are P. Ekman, "Are there basic emotions?" *Psychological Review* 99 (1992): 550–553; and P. Ekman, *Darwin and Facial Expression: A Century of Research in Review.* New York: Academic Press, 1973.

8. Initially they were asked to pick the posed emotion from six words from their own language, but this procedure was soon abandoned because of the linguistic uncertainty about the words matching the emotion. Not only were there uncertainties about translation; different cultures may have differing relations between language and states of mind. So they constructed very simple narratives to allow the New Guineans to understand an emotional response, for example, you are angry and about to fight, or your child has died.

9. D. Buss, "Is there a universal human nature?" *Contemporary Psychology* 37 (1992): 1262–1263.

10. A. Ortony, and T. J. Taylor, "What's basic about basic emotions?" *Psychological Review* 97 (1990): 315–331.

11. J. Panksepp, "Toward a general psychobiological theory of emotions," *The Behavioral and Brain Sciences* 5 (1982): 407–467.

12. J. A. Gray, *The Neuropsychology of Anxiety.* Oxford: Oxford University Press, 1982.

13. R. Plutchik, *The Emotions: Facts, Theories, and a New Model.* New York: Random House, 1962.

14. See P. Ekman, "Strong evidence for universals in facial expression: A reply to Russell's mistaken critique," *Psychological Bulletin* 115 (1994): 268–287; and C. E. Izard, "Innate and universal facial expression: Evidence from developmental and cross-cultural research," *Psychological Bulletin* 115 (1994): 288–299.

15. A. J. Fridlund, "Evolution and facial action in reflex, social motive and paralanguage," *Biological Psychology* 32 (1991): 3–100.

16. In Darwin's account the display arose from association with the emotion underlying the act, a far more tortuous and difficult route to understand (or accept). The third source of facial display is its association with language, so-called facial paralanguage.

17. Bell and Darwin agreed that some facial movements arose in association with respiration. Ekman and Friesen classified fewer than one third of the facial actions of patients during psychiatric interviews as being "emotional." P. Ekman, and W. V. Friesen, Unpublished. Cited in P. Ekman, Biological and cultural contributions to body and facial movement. In J. Blacking (Ed.), *The Anthropology of the Body.* London: Academic Press, 1977. It is not known how skewed the result was because the patients were suffering from affective disorders.

18. I am grateful to the anonymous MIT reader for suggesting this consideration of Fridlund's work.

19. To look at nonhuman primates in this way assumes some common origin for us and the other nonhuman primates, which seems reasonably secure, even though we split from them several million years ago, and have been engaged in parallel evolution since, with extinction of many of our nearer cousins.

20. J. A. R. A. M. Van Hooff, "The facial displays of catarrhine monkeys and apes." In *Primate Ethology,* edited by D. Morris. London: Weidenfeld & Nicholson, 1967. Others who have delineated facial displays include Jane Goodall, *The Chimpanzees of Gombe: Patterns of Behavior.* Cambridge, MA: Harvard University Press, 1986; and Alison Jolly, *The Evolution of Primate Behaviour.* London, Macmillan, 1985.

21. In their natural environment direct gaze is threatening, unless the two individuals know each other or one or both are immature, but this is not necessarily the case in captive chimpanzees. In one of her books Jane Goodall describes direct eye contact with a chimp. A former student of hers, Alison Alp, wrote to me from Sierra Leone, where she was studying chimpanzees, that there was one captive chimp, Bruno, who when praised would sit gazing at her face for as long as she talked to him.

22. A similar idea had come by letter from Jonathan Kingdon, a member of the animal ethology research group at Oxford. I had asked him if there were less well-known, poorly decoded facial displays which might need more idiosyncratic interpretation by others. He replied that in evolutionary terms there might have been a need for a "cut-off" from challenges and communications that were energy draining and potentially damaging. Facial expression, tied in with social repertoire, expended energy and so cutting them out might conserve it. In this context "blank negative expressions might be interesting as well as positive ones."

23. The orangs were at the refuge because they are used by photographers in Taiwan.

24. R. W. Burn, and Andrew Whiten, In *Natural Theories of Mind: Evolution, Development and Simulation of Everyday Mindreading,* edited by Andrew Whiten. Oxford: Blackwell, 1991.

25. G. Gallup, "Self-awareness and the emergence of mind in primates," *American Journal of Primatology* 2 (1982): 237–248.

26. In Freud's *New Introductory Lectures on Psychoanalysis* (London: Penguin Books, 1973), the index goes from "External World (see Reality)," to "Faeces, equated with baby and penis," with no mention of "face."

Chapter 6

1. J. C. Gomez, Visual behaviour as a window for reading the minds of others in primates. In *Natural Theories of Mind; Evolution, Development and Simulation of Everyday Mindreading,* edited by Andrew Whiten. Oxford: Blackwell, 1991.

2. That perception of gaze direction is important might be inferred by the fact that in humans, unlike in most primates, the whites of our eyes show, allowing others to see clearly where, and at what, we are looking. (See Butterworth, G. "The ontology and phylogeny of joint visual attention." In Andrew Whiten, op. cit., 1991).

3. D. Premack, and G. Woodruff, "Does the chimpanzee have a 'theory of mind?'" *Behavior and Brain Sciences* 4 (1978): 515–526.

4. Some evidence suggests not. See S. Baron-Cohen, *Mindblindness* (Cambridge, MA: The MIT Press, 1995, pp. 121–125), for a review.

5. H. Wimmer, and J. Perner, "Belief about beliefs: Representation and constraining function of wrong beliefs in young children's understanding of deception," *Cognition* 13 (1983): 103–128.

6. S. Baron-Cohen, A. Leslie, and U. Frith, "Does the autistic child have a 'theory of mind?'" *Cognition* 21 (1985): 37–46. For a fuller description of the literature on theory of mind see S. Baron-Cohen, H. Tager-Flusberg, and D. J. Cohen, *Understanding Other Minds, Perspectives from Autism.* Oxford: Oxford Medical Publications, 1993.

7. A. M. Leslie, "Pretense and representation: The origins of 'theory of mind,'" *Psychological Review* 94 (1987): 412–426.

8. J. Perner, *Understanding the Representational Mind.* Cambridge, MA: The MIT Press, 1990.

9. Similar ideas have been discussed in portraiture for many years; see E. H. Gombrich, "The mask and the face: The perception of physiognomic likeness in life and art." In *Art, Perception and Reality,* edited by E. H. Gombrich, J. Hochberg, and M. Black, 1–46. Baltimore: Johns Hopkins University Press, 1972. It may also have resonances in acting, for how can I portray anyone accurately, by acting or by imagining myself in that position, by aping actions or by experiencing them and so by way of a theory of mind, understanding the other?

10. S. Baron-Cohen, *Mindblindness.* Cambridge, MA: The MIT Press, 1994. For a criticism, see D. J. Povinelli, and T. J. Povinelli, *Trends in the Neurosciences* 19 (1996): 299–300.

11. He illustrates the model with diagrams of the areas of the brain that may be involved in this, suggesting that the eye direction detector may be in the superior temporal sulcus and the amygdala, and the theory of mind mechanism in the orbito-frontal cortex, that is, the ventromedial part of the frontal lobe.

12. R. P Hobson, *Autism and the Development of Mind.* Hillsdale, NJ: Erlbaum, 1993.

13. D. N. Stern, *The First Relationship, Infant and Mother.* Cambridge, MA: Harvard University Press, 1977.

14. D. N. Stern, *The Interpersonal World of the Infant.* New York: Basic Books, 1985.

15. L. Kanner, "Autistic disturbance of affective contact," *Nervous Child* 2 (1943): 217–250.

16. H. Asperger, "Die 'autistischen Psychopathen' in Kindesalter," *Archiv für Psychiatrie and Nervenkrankenheiten* 117 (1944): 76–136. For an English translation, see U. Frith, ed., *Autism and Asperger Syndrome.* Cambridge: Cambridge University Press, 1991.

17. Oliver Sacks, *An Anthropologist on Mars.* New York: Knopf, 1995.

18. See, for example; Clara Claiborne Park, *The Seige: The First Eight Years of an Autistic Child.* London: Pelican Books, 1967. Paperback edition, London: Pelican Books, 1972. In Frith, *Autism and Asperger Syndrome,* Cambridge: Cambridge University Press, 1991, there are several accounts of people with autism and Asperger syndrome, including an analysis of autobiographical writings by Francesca Happé. See also Temple Grandin, and M. M. Scariano, *Emergence Labelled Autistic* . Novato, CA: Arena Press, 1986.

19. "I disagree. Asperger's can speak easier 'in the world' [language, writing], but some able autistic people, can, with big effort, 'speak with pictures.'" (I showed this chapter and, of course, the next to Donna Williams, an extraordinarily gifted person with a form of autism. She offered some comments, which I have included in the notes in quotation marks.)

20. Donna Williams's suggestion.

21. F. R. Volmar, "Social development." In *Handbook of Autism,* edited by D. Cohen and A. Donnelan, 41–60. New York: Wiley, 1987.

22. C. Delacato, *The Ultimate Stranger.* New York: Doubleday, 1974, cited in Stella Carlton, *The Other Side of Autism,* Worcester, UK: The Self-Publishing Association, 1993.

23. Grandin and Scariano, *Emergence Labeled Autistic,* pp. 22–23. Novato, CA: Arena Press, 1986.

24. Though for Donna Williams communication through monologue is possible.

25. M. Rutter, and E. Schopler, "Autism and pervasive developmental disorders," *Journal of Autism and Developmental Disorders* 17 (1987): 159–186.

26. By rote learning rather than in a context.

27. S. Baron-Cohen, A. Spitz, and P. Cross, "Can children with autism recognize surprise?" *Cognition and Emotion* 7 (1993): 507–516.

28. At the school I went to there was a boy nicknamed "Mong" (short for Mongol, an insensitive term formerly used for persons with Down syndrome and hence for developmental problems as well). The school was a grammar school and one had to pass a quite stiff entrance exam, so the boys were quite academic. But Mong was known throughout the school for his ineptitude. He was as useless at games as at social interaction, and had a habit of staring at the floor when you talked to him. His claim to fame was that he had memorized the positions in the pop charts for each week for every record over the previous twenty years. I have no idea if he was diagnosed and helped.

29. "This man's visual processing was 'on-line' here. For others visual processing may be like the system that gives way as a compensation in response to overload. For others it may be auditory processing, emotional processing, or body connectedness or a swing between each—that is, systems shifts in 'mono' processing." (Donna describes her inability to be connected with more than one perceptual system at once as being mono.)

30. "Here there is a self-other 'mono,' but this not necessarily a lack of perception (outside of social context) of other minds."

31. "In immediate context I and many assume that others must think or feel the same because there is no thought otherwise to the contrary—so it is the only assumption possible."

32. "or be aware of feeling?"

33. "i.e., because it may not be being processed."

34. Jonathan Cole, *Pride and a Daily Marathon* Cambridge, MA: The MIT Press, 1995.

35. "trying to function as multi-track when he is essentially 'mono.'"

36. "Lucky multitrack non-auties."

37. "body on line fulfilling a rote-learned task."

38. "thought, verbal accessing and auditory processing on-line."

39. "Maybe she creates less 'other' impact so the self-other balance required is more manageable."

40. "You do not have self/other mono, you are multi track and maintain both SIMULTANEOUSLY, consistently."

41. "Echolalia and echopraxia are not about feeling but about the disconnected expression."

42. "who could not hold consistently simultaneous sense of self and other."

43. "in the context they occurred as they occurred."

Chapter 7

1. Donna Williams, *Nobody Nowhere*. New York: Random, London: Corgi Books, 1992.

2. Donna Williams, *Somebody Somewhere*. New York: Random, London: Corgi Books, 1994.

3. The italics here are Donna's comments on my draft MS. She read all parts of the book concerned with autism. The form of Donna Williams's autistic disorder has remained controversial since the publication of her first book. Her exceptional insight and gifts have even led some to doubt the diagnosis. In person, however, she has characteristics common to those with autistic disorder. Her insights seem compatible with behavior observed in persons with autism, and so her insights have been included in the present work.

4. Remember Oliver Sacks's description of the individuality of people with autism and Asperger syndrome, and in this they are no different from the rest of us. Donna's experiences may not be typical of other people with autism. The fact that she has an extraordinary ability to communicate through monologue takes her beyond many with autism.

5. "Of surviving in a harsh environment trying to 'act normal.'"

6. "without fear of losing control of the interaction and the experience and feelings it caused."

7. In an earlier draft I had written not "someone," but "friend" she had met in the park. She corrected me. "No friends."

8. "I knew factually that people cried in response to your words if they'd been impacted upon."

9. "but it was, with reduction in other forms of overload, becoming easier to process and, therefore, more tolerable."

10. In an earlier draft I had written, "in particular seek to help a young autistic girl." Donna wrote, "I did NOT 'seek to help.' I was being with. I had a great empathy for her *as* me, not as a separate person. 'Seek to help' is 'the world' speak and is not appropriate in this context." Guilty as charged, I found it difficult reading her prose, not to impose my meaning, *our* meaning, on her experience and actions. It concerns me therefore that her books, though so bright and clear, may still be capable of being misinterpreted by "non-auties."

11. "Echopraxia has nothing to do with understanding—quite the reverse."

12. "in adapting to functioning in a predominantly non-autistic world."

13. "with the exception of the feedback her own automatic, preconscious writing gave her."

14. "self, meaning with intent."

15. Oliver Sacks, *An Anthropologist on Mars.* New York: Knopf, 1995.

16. "Only if that other has such a weak sense of imposing self is it possible for the other not to cause cut off from self."

17. "Wish something was—my conscious mind is like a blocked toilet."

18. It was clear that Donna and Paul were trying to find meaning in bewildering extravagances of sensory input and image. In complete contrast, Bacon, happy in and with his perceptions of reality and imagination, sought to extend and distort in order to reveal and express feeling.

Chapter 8

1. J. Piaget, *Play, dreams and imitation in childhood.* New York: Norton, 1962.

2. A. Meltzoff, and M. K. Moore, "Imitation of facial and manual gestures by human neonates." *Science* 198 (1977): 75–78.

3. I. W. R. Bushnell, F. Sai, and J. T. Mullin, "Neonatal recognition of the mother's face." *British Journal of Developmental Psychology* 7 (1989): 3–15.

4. A. Meltzoff, and M. K. Moore, "Early imitation within a functional framework; the importance of person identity, movement and development." *Infant Behavior and Development* 15 (1992): 479–505.

5. A. N. Meltzoff, and M. K. Moore, "Why faces are special to infants—on connecting the attraction of faces and infants' ability for imitation and cross modal processing." In *Developmental Neurocognition: Speech and Face Processing in the First Year of Life,* edited by B. Boysson-Bardies et al., 211–225. Dordecht: Kluwer Academic Publishers, 1993.

6. A. Meltzoff, and A. Gopnik, "The role of imitation in understanding persons and developing a theory of mind." In *Understanding Other Minds,* edited by S. Baron-Cohen, H. Tager-Flusberg, and D. J. Cohen. Oxford: Oxford University Press, 1993.

7. There are theories of how emotion may have evolved and of its physiological basis and role, with varying degrees of empirical evidence (see, e.g., Michael Lewis and Linda Michelson, Faces as signs and symbols. In *The Development of Expressive Behavior,* edited by Gail Zivin. Orlando, FL: Academic Press, 1985). The problem is not in the development of theories but in their testing, for this is an extraordinarily difficult area to provide hard data in. Lewis and Michelson approach this matter from a slightly different perspective. They suggest that initially a baby's facial expression is not related to internal emotional states. As emotional development occurs the baby integrates the two. Then, later, social pressures force it to learn to dissociate expression from internal states as the baby becomes sophisticated and non-naive.

8. D. N. Stern, *The First Relationship, Infant and Mother.* Cambridge, MA: Harvard University Press, 1977.

9. D. N. Stern, *The Interpersonal World of the Infant.* New York: Basic Books, 1985.

10. This may start even before birth. My wife, when carrying our daughters, would often go off at a meeting or party and sit on her own, with an inner beatific look; she was engaging with her child. That same look would often be there when feeding or just when she was with our young babies.

11. Anthony Manstead, and Roselyne Edwards, "Communicative aspects of children's emotional competence." In *International Review of Studies of Emotion,* edited by K. T. Strongman. New York: Wiley, 1992.

12. There are, of course, social factors involved in the rules of engagement through gaze which involve, among other things, culture, seniority, and social class. These are not my concern here.

13. Edmund Burke and Charles Bell considered this, the latter writing, ". . . by the actions and expressions of the body betraying the passions of the heart we may be startled and forewarned, as it were, by the reflection of ourselves, and at the same time learn to control our passions by restraining the expression of them." Charles Bell, *Essays on the Anatomy and Philosophy of Expression,* 3rd rev. ed. London: John Murray, 1844.

14. "[W]hen the actor properly imitates all the external signs . . . and all the bodily alterations which . . . are expressions of a particular [inner] state, the resulting impression will automatically induce a state in his soul that properly accords with his own movements, posture and vocal tone." (Gotthold Lessing, quoted in A. J. Fridlund, "Evolution and facial action in reflex, social motive and paralanguage," *Biological Psychology* 32 (1991): 3–100.)

15. There is some dispute about Darwin's precise aims in this passage. Some have placed it in the context of a facial feedback model, in which facial expression modifies inner states. In contrast, Fridlund suggested simply that Darwin was pointing out that loss of control may follow an excessive emotional outburst. Charles Darwin, *The Expression of the Emotions in Men and Animals*. Chicago: University of Chicago Press, 1965.

16. William James, *The Principles of Psychology*. 2 vols. New York: Dover, 1950.

17. A. J. Fridlund, "Evolution and facial action in reflex, social motive and paralanguage," *Biological Psychology* 32 (1991): 3–100.

18. P. K. Adelman, and R. B. Zajonc, "Facial efference and emotion," *Annual Review of Psychology* 40 (1989): 249–280.

19. D. Goldblatt, and D. Williams, "'I Am Smiling!' Möbius syndrome inside and out," *Journal of Child Psychology and Psychiatry and Allied Disciplines* 1 (1986): 71–78. I am grateful to Colin Brennan for bringing this article and much more about Möbius to my attention.

Chapter 9

1. There is debate as to the extent to which some people with Möbius are of borderline low intelligence. In one series of sixteen cases from Great Ormond Street Hospital five were of low intelligence with a further three difficult to assess (Peter Bannister, Jane Walker, and Kenneth Wybar, "Möbius's syndrome," *British Orthoptics Journal* 33 (1976): 69–77). Two were initially thought to be low but then later were considered to have normal or high IQ levels. The author commented that milestones of even those with normal intelligence are delayed, so assessment is difficult, especially since IQ is related to age. As Meyerson and Foushee have pointed out, the delays in development in children with Möbius may be unsurprising given the enormity of their handicaps, which may involve foot and hand deformity, squint, and poor growth because of feeding difficulties, let alone the problems associated with speech and emotional expression and interaction. To my knowledge there has not been a series of tests in children plotting IQ against time to show if they start slowly and then catch up. See M. D. Meyerson, and D. R. Fousheen, "Speech, language and hearing in Möbius syndrome: A study of 22 patients," *Developmental Medicine and Child Neurology* 20 (1987): 357–365.

2. I am happy that Clare felt herself to belong to a group. Yet people with Möbius look similar to untutored eyes in the way that Chinese all tend to look alike to whites, and vice versa. When known, the individuality becomes apparent. Some people with Möbius remind me facially of some of Modigliani's portraits, especially *The Little Milkmaid,* with her blank eyes. When we blink, the eyes roll upward in their sockets (first described by Charles Bell, and known as Bell's phenomenon). Normally this is not seen since the eyelids are shut at the time. In subjects with Möbius the lids do not move, and so it is seen. This "lidless blink" has a curious interrupting effect on conversation since the persons appears to absent himself or herself from your presence during it.

3. There is some evidence that touching of the face increases with phylogenetic development of the face itself. The more facially mobile and expressive higher monkeys and apes caress and feel their own faces more, with humans doing it the most. At meetings with colleagues I often look around the room and at any one time about half those present are stroking their faces absent mindedly or touching them in various ways.

4. James had said that he had difficulty in the street knowing if people were going to speak to him. People with Möbius may not learn to read others' faces very well. Their difficulty in moving the eyes makes looking at people a stare, which is awkward. Their feelings of low esteem make it less likely that they would approach others; looking at someone to enter into a conversation requires courage. So by turning from their own faces they may not attend to others.' In addition, by not elaborating their own facial expression they may be less aware of its importance to others, and be less able to interpret emotion in others. James said that he not been a student of other people's faces until recently.

5. For a consideration of these matters of feelings and intellect and more see Antonio Damasio, *Descartes' Error.* New York: Grosset/Putnam, 1994, especially chapter 11.

6. The facial feedback hypothesis suggested that we do not simply smile when we are happy, but rather, in its extreme version, that we are happy when we smile; that the feedback from our faces determines mood. Some ingenious experiments in control subjects have provided evidence for this, though one might say that feedback consolidates and reinforces rather than determines emotional states. People with Möbius have lived a cruel experiment on this matter from birth. Their experience reveals the effects of absent facial movement on emotional development, social interaction, and sense of self far more eloquently than any short experiment.

Chapter 10

1. Sarcoid is a common cause of bilateral Bell's palsy.

2. Oliver Sacks in *A Leg to Stand On* (New York: Summit, 1984) considers some of the difficulties in recovering movement following immobility. In his case it was a leg, but the same may well be as, or more, relevant to the face.

3. Brian Keenan, *An Evil Cradling.* London: Hutchinson, 1992.

4. Oliver Sacks, *Awakenings.* New York: Harper Perennial, 1990.

5. Fortunately, her eyelid was not open permanently, or she would have needed a pad over it or a suture in the lid to protect the eye itself.

6. Facial features depend on the skin and the muscles that move the face. As we have seen, these are well attached to the bones and, with the years, they can sag. Apart from moving the face, they also have a resting tone, which is destroyed in Bell's palsy. In Brenda the tone or posture of the facial muscles was increasing as a result of the disordered regrowth of the facial nerve. She felt this overactivity of the

facial muscles at rest as a tightness. The cause for this was not inactivity in the facial nerve. Following Bell's palsy the facial nerve had regrown and was firing at a low level continually and uncontrollably, altering the resting posture of the face and making it feel and look different. The problem now was, paradoxically, not paralysis but overactivity.

7. This was caused by aberrant regrowth of nerve fibers in the facial nerve. Some are known to branch within the nerve trunk in the face. Normally the branching allows a given nerve to control firing of several muscle fibers in one part of the face, for example, around the mouth, the nose, or the upper or lower part of the eye. After damage to the nerve there can be branching to both mouth and eye. Then a command to move the eye can also lead to mouth movement, a phenomenon known as synkinesis. It usually fades with time, but in this case, possibly because of the chaotic nerve damage and regrowth, it was more persistent and prolonged.

8. Young chimpanzees are also allowed to stare at their elders.

9. Interestingly, it was by thinking through her feelings that she came to this conclusion. As a doctor or healthcare worker one is taught not to allow feelings so near the surface. As soon as you do become too interested, and feelings enter into the observation, then you may be no longer acting purely professionally, but humanely.

10. *Face to Face: Parkinson's Disease—Facial Animation Made Easier.* Parkinson's Disease Society videocassette, 1993. It is available from Iona Lister, Speech and Language Therapy, Horton General Hospital, Banbury, Oxon, OX16 9AL, United Kingdom.

11. Iona got some ideas from a cheap video about how to stay young in which a woman contends that faces look old and decrepit because we allow gravity to take over and our faces to drop.

Chapter 11

1. James Partridge, *Changing Faces*. London: Penguin, 1990.

Chapter 12

1. D. R. Rubinow, and R. M. Post, "Impaired recognition of affect in facial expression in depressed patients." *Biological Psychiatry* 31 (1992): 947–953.

2. J. Archer, D.C. Hay, and A. W. Young, "Face processing in psychiatric conditions," *British Journal of Clinical Psychology* 31 (1992): 45–61.

3. Alison told me of one man sent to such a place as a boy. His parents were the gatekeepers of a large house. Their master had made them commit him because he had a cleft lip and was unsightly to visitors.

4. At a meeting kindly arranged by Bencie Woll. She, incidentally, has begun to look at grammatical and emotional use of the face in signers.

5. Recall that one of the advantages in the "facialization" of body language in pri-

mates was that the face could be directed in space toward a person far more than the body could. This is taken a stage further with eye movements and mutual gaze.

6. Bruno Bettelheim spoke of the autistic person as being constantly in jeopardy.

7. If the face is so important for "self-other" balance, how remarkable then that in psychoanalysis, which is so concerned with these balances, the face is not studied.

8. Ludwig Wittgenstein, *Remarks on the Philosophy of Psychology*. Chicago: University of Chicago Press, 1980.

9. R. P. Hobson, *Autism and the Development of Mind*. Hillsdale, NJ: Erlbaum, 1993.

10. Nicholas Humphrey, *The Inner Eye*. London: Faber & Faber, 1986.

11. R. I. M. Dunbar, "Ecological modelling in an evolutionary context," *Folia Primatologica (Basel)* 53 (1990): 235–246. (Quoted in Merlin Donald, *Origins of the Modern Mind*. Cambridge, MA: Harvard University Press, 1993.)

12. In extrapolating these data to humans, Merlin Donald estimated the group size for those six surviving aboriginal societies, which are nomadic or hunter-gatherer, and then compared human and primate brain size with the numbers in their social groups. He predicted an ideal human group size of 223, and found an average size in hunters of 156 and nomads of 174. Chimpanzees, by contrast, may know forty or so fellow chimps. Compare this number with the vast number of people we see now. Trying to predict behavior in people hardly known may be one reason for the use of physiognomy and astrology. Both try to find general rules for personality from dubious data. Both are doomed to failure.

13. There may be a relationship between nonhuman primates' facial expressivity, their social group stability, and intelligence. Facial mobility in humans may be linked to perceived intelligence. As women have become more accepted as intellectual equals, there has been an increasing acceptance of older women's beauty. Mature women naturally have more expressive and mobile faces than younger women, who are often cast in a more passive role.

14. In this I have been exclusively concerned with terrestrial animals with vision as a dominant sense. It is possible that the large aquatic mammals have developed some parallel system through, say, vocalization. To suggest that the congenitally deaf or blind develop normal awareness of self and others despite their sensory losses is to miss the point, for their brains have evolved to have those senses. The relevant question is what sort of world and consciousness of self and others would develop in successive generations of blind or deaf individuals? This is similarly unknowable to what sort of existence would Möbius subjects have experienced if they had grown up in a world of blind people.

15. Antonio Damasio, *Descartes' Error: Emotion, Reason and the Human Brain*. New York: Putnam, 1995.

16. Politics may be a fascinating example of this. Reagan and Thatcher, for good or ill, were never slow in coming to decisions. They were driven by conviction, and so imposed their political values, their likes and dislikes, their gut instincts, on their actions. Clinton and Major had reputations for being indecisive and vacillating

in part because they try to see all sides of an argument and reach decisions more cerebrally and rationally.

17. I have not stressed the work suggesting that feedback of emotion arises from these autonomic organs. In part because one must be careful, for much of this feedback is preconscious. It is the selective aspects of this, the sinking feeling in the stomach with a shock, or the tightening with nerves that we do perceive. In addition, this feedback does not appear to be very subtle emotionally, nor, with the exception of blushing, is it communicated.

18. William James, *The Principles of Psychology,* 2 vols. 1890. Reprint New York: Dover, 1950.

19. In such a group of people it is almost impossible to distinguish the problems associated with their psychiatric condition from those arising from their social deprivation. A most extreme example of this arises very infrequently: so-called feral children, who have grown up without human company. Zingg, in a historical study of thirty-one such children, gave no good description of their use of facial displays, nor was there one in the work of Itard, a French physician who tried to rehabilitate the Wild Boy of Aveyron. Feral children, however, do show a limited range of expressive behavior such as anger, joy, depression, and impatience, but their appropriateness has always been very difficult to establish because of their asocial behavior and rapid mood shifts. The most famous case, Kaspar Hauser, who was incarcerated, was considered to have suffered a "crime against the human soul." See R. M. Zingg, "Feral man and extreme cases of isolation," *American Journal of Psychology* 53 (1940): 487–517; and J. Itard, *The Wild Boy of Aveyron.* New York: Appleton, 1932.

20. Peter Hobson, personal communication, 1995.

21. Donna Williams, Personal communication, 1995.

22. Emmanuel Levinas, *Collected Philosophical Papers.* Dordrecht, Netherlands: Kluwer. I am grateful to Shaun Gallagher of Canisius College, New York, for introducing me to Levinas's writing and for guiding me through it. Levinas died in 1996.

23. Maurice Merleau-Ponty, *The Primacy of Perception.* Evanston, IL: Northwestern University Press, 1964.

24. Charles Bell, *Essays on the Anatomy and Philosophy of Expression,* 2nd ed. London: John Murray, 1824.

25. Peter Brook once described the theater as allowing us "to look at those we would otherwise condemn or walk past" (in a discussion with Ian Waterman and David Bennent about the play *The Man Who).* In other words, art may allow us to enter the minds and experiences of others and to attempt to understand those who otherwise would be foreign. While in some parts of this book I have discussed science, I have mostly been concerned with narratives of people in exceptional circumstances, and related these narratives in a manner not usually thought of as scientific. Luria suggested that his great neuropsychological biographies (*Man with a Shattered World* and *The Mind of a Mnemonist),* were "romantic science," but that seems an unfortunate term. "Human-based science" is clumsy. But whatever it is called, the entering into the experience of others through listening to their stories

seemed a most important way to investigate what the face means. Francis Bacon wrote, "the greatest art will always bring you back to the vulnerability of the human situation." It is from those in whom the natural flow of life is not present—Bacon's "vulnerable," Brook's "walked past"—that we can learn much about the human situation and about face.

26. Anchee Min, *Red Azalea*. London: Victor Gollancz, 1993.

27. John Liggett, *The Human Face*. London: Constable, 1974.

Index